Praise for
Energy Healing for Animals

"Joan Ranquet knows a lot about energy and a lot about animals. From her creative synthesis of these two passions, you are the beneficiary, empowered to elevate the physical and emotional well-being of the animals you love. This book brings you into a mindset that will help you resonate with your pets while providing practical techniques for getting desired results."

DONNA EDEN
author of *Energy Medicine*

"For the last couple of decades, a phone call to Joan is the first thing I do when I have issues with my pets. She is a most compassionate and intuitive healer, with an uncanny ability to zero in on what's ailing them."

JANE LYNCH
actress and animal advocate

"Anything you've ever wanted to know to enhance the health and happiness of animals can be found in *Energy Healing for Animals*. Joan Ranquet's knowledge, wisdom, and experience with animals is rounded out with explanations of modalities, techniques, science, and practices of vibrational healing—and much more. Get your highlighter ready! You will want this book for your library. Very impressive."

MARGARET ANN LEMBO
author of *Chakra Awakening: Transform Your Reality Using Crystals, Color, Aromatherapy and the Power of Positive Thought*

"I know Joan Ranquet to be a master animal healer, trainer, teacher, and communicator. I have the greatest love and respect for her unusual gifts and talents.

Joan's voracious quest for healing has led her to the very best practices of 2,000 years of human energy healing, which has only gone mainstream in the last 30 years. Because of her special bond and gifts with our four-legged, winged, and even finned animal friends, Joan has taken 2,000 years of healing wisdom and adapted it for our most beloved animal companions.

I once heard healing with energy medicine described as simply 'giving love.' Animals, with their capacity for unconditional love, often respond far better than humans to energy treatments. Joan's new book, *Energy Healing for Animals*, is crystal clear in its writing and teaching. It allows any two-legged human to easily learn these time-tested energy medicine techniques and 'share love' with all your beloveds. I highly recommend it to you."   ALAN DAVIDSON

creator of Enlightened Tapping,
founder of ThroughYourBody.com,
author of *Body Brilliance: Mastering Your Five Vital Intelligences*

"Everything you've ever needed to know about energy healing for the precious souls that journey the earth with us—animals—is here in Joan Ranquet's book, *Energy Healing for Animals*. As an energy practitioner and long-time companion animal owner, I've needed a book like this for decades. Like us, animals are composed of a series of energy systems. How can I use love, intention, and 'emotional leadership,' one of Joan's key phrases, to balance and support the animals in my world? How about energy techniques, nutrition, and telepathy? Every tool is here in the book that can change the way we perceive and bond with our animals."   CYNDI DALE

author of *The Subtle Body*

"Joan Ranquet's love for animals shines through on every page of this carefully crafted and thought-provoking book. She has left no stone unturned as she explains the myriad of healing modalities available for dogs, cats, and horses. From the mundane (nutrition) to the more esoteric (Reiki), her descriptions are clear, thorough, and engaging. Save yourself time, heartache, and frequent trips to the vet by getting a copy of this book! I know I will be referring to *Energy Healing for Animals* again and again. I now have a user-friendly, treasured set of new tools at my disposal to create health, wellness, and happiness among the animals in my household. Thank you, Joan!"

MEADOW LINN
author of *The Mystic Cookbook: The Secret Alchemy of Food*

"There is nothing more important to me—more precious to my heart—than my beloved dogs. They are in every way to me my children. There is nothing I would not do for them—nothing I would not give them to ensure their happiness, well-being, and safety. After 30 years of working within the spiritual and metaphysical world, I have experienced many healers and intuitives. And in all of that time I have never come across anyone as gifted, in tune, and connected to the animal kingdom as Joan Ranquet. She has conversed with every 'four-pawed child' of my adult life with undeniable accuracy. The result has been happier and longer lives for all of them.

And now Joan has brought all of her knowledge, experience, and spiritual gifts together into the creation of *Energy Healing for Animals*. Inside these pages you will find insights into the animal kingdom that will surprise, delight, and amaze you. If you love animals, then you know in your heart that their souls are akin to your own. Let Joan give you the tools necessary to glimpse deeply into their world and discover just how right you are about that."

RADLEIGH VALENTINE
bestselling Hay House author,
spiritual teacher, and radio show host.

"Since I met Joan when she helped me locate a lost pet, I've been consistently impressed with her insights and skills. As a veterinarian practicing integrative medicine, I find her new book, *Energy Healing for Animals*, to be illuminating as she shares her experiences that have taken her to learning about guiding energy techniques. Her goal of harvesting the correct energy paths to maximize health and happiness is inspirational and makes it easy to refocus when any patient/pet is in need. I know those who read this will find themselves equally engrossed in the pages."
CINDY RIGG, DVM, CCRT
cindyriggdvm.com

"The thing about energy healing is that you do it all the time whether you realize it or not. So you may as well learn a thing or two, and this is a great place to start! Nice overview and entertaining—but don't underestimate the powerful insight and tips Joan gives from a lifetime of deepening wisdom by communicating with all life."
DR. PENNY LLOYD
veterinarian, ConnectionMedicine.com

"*Energy Healing for Animals* is a delightful, beautifully written book. Once you witness its applications, you will know why this is a must-have book for healing. What Joan teaches is a must for anyone wanting lasting health for their beloved pets."
DR. FRANK BOUSAID
holistic veterinarian, Harmony Animal
Wellness Clinic, hawcmonroe.com

"*Energy Healing for Animals* is a cornucopia of emotional and physical support and loving healing methods you can offer your beloved animals. There's so much you can do to have happy, healthy companion animals. Just delve into *Energy Healing for Animals* and you will learn so much about animal communication, chakras, acupressure, bodywork, and so much more—all to benefit animals! Joan Ranquet set out to provide a healing toolbox for us to enjoy with our animals, and that she did."
AMY SNOW & NANCY ZIDONIS
authors and founders of Tallgrass Animal Acupressure Institute

"This book is truly a master class in cutting-edge healing modalities, teaching how to both heal and shift the behavior of the animal you love. Joan Ranquet has taken a broad field of approaches and clarified, simplified, and assembled them into an incredible resource and how-to book filled with her rich wisdom. This practical dive into energy, vibrational frequencies, emotional leadership, and intention will surely transform you as you bring a new level of healing and connection to the treasured animals in your life."

MARGARET LYNCH
author of *Tapping into Wealth*, success mentor,
and premier EFT® teacher

"After seeing Joan in action personally, I am a true fan of hers. Having the ability to communicate with animals myself, I now have the tools to improve my skills with Joan's newest book, *Energy Healing for Animals*. Everything I need to know to communicate with the animals in my life is contained in this gem!"

MADISYN TAYLOR
DailyOM

"A potent offering . . . affirming that love and the intention we hold in our heart is the basis of all healing. Thank you, Joan, for your service in the world."

LINDA BENDER, DVM
author of *Animal Wisdom:
Learning from the Spiritual Lives of Animals*

"I love this book. It belongs in the collection of every person interested in the merging of quantum science, spirituality, and healing. Whether you are a newbie to the concept of healing animals with energy or thoroughly acquainted with the possibilities that exist when we recognize the healing power of thought, emotion, and vibration—you will find a treasure trove in this integration of ancient concepts of energy with the latest understanding of quantum science. I give it five stars!"

LINDA TELLINGTON-JONES, PHD
founder and president of Tellington TTouch™ Training

"With respect, passion, and compassion for the animals, and humorous professional experiences, Ms. Ranquet is a natural storyteller as she guides us through vibrational healing techniques to soothe all of our souls. From chakras to tapping, quantum physics resonance to flower essences, Joan Ranquet's *Energy Healing for Animals* shows us how these techniques work with and through the animals, giving animal guardians efficient, unique tools for the 21st century. A great offering to four-legged well-being."   CHERYL SCHWARTZ, DVM
holistic healer and author of *Four Paws, Five Directions:*
A Guide to Chinese Medicine for Cats and Dogs
and *Natural Healing for Dogs and Cats A–Z*

Energy Healing *for* Animals

*A Hands-On Guide for Enhancing the Health,
Longevity & Happiness of Your Pets*

JOAN RANQUET

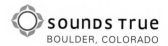

BOULDER, COLORADO

Sounds True
Boulder, CO 80306

This work is solely for personal growth and education. It should not be treated as a substitute for professional assistance, therapeutic activities, or medical advice. In the event of physical or mental distress, please consult with appropriate health professionals. The application of protocols and information in this book is the choice of each reader, who assumes full responsibility for his or her understandings, interpretations, and results. The author and publisher assume no responsibility for the actions or choices of any reader.

Published 2015

Cover design by Lisa Kerans
Book design by Beth Skelley

Printed in the United States of America

Library of Congress Cataloging-in-Publication Data
  Ranquet, Joan.
  Energy healing for animals : a hands-on guide for enhancing the health,
  longevity, and happiness of your pets / Joan Ranquet.
     pages cm
  Includes bibliographical references.
  ISBN 978-1-60407-671-4
  1. Alternative veterinary medicine. 2. Energy medicine. I. Title.
  SF745.5.R365 2015
  636.089'55—dc23
                          2015014220

Ebook ISBN 978-1-60407-757-5

10 9 8 7 6 5 4 3 2 1

This book is dedicated to all the animals that have dared to incarnate in time to live with me! It's also dedicated to all the animals I have been lucky enough to communicate with and facilitate healing for. And it is dedicated to all the people who trusted me enough to pick up the phone or to go to my website and give this work a chance.

Contents

Introduction:
Connecting With Animals

As a young child, I had something like an obsessive-compulsive disorder. Whenever an animal got close to me, I just had to look into its eyes. It was as if I were registering every creature's existence in a giant record book somewhere. This was especially true for the meekest of beings. As I looked into their eyes, I fell into a sea of compassion. You could say that I've never climbed out of the water.

Three things hold true for me with animals: I can't not look at them, I can't avoid truly seeing them, and I can't avoid acknowledging them.

This is who I am. They are a part of me. Connecting with animals is my gift, and early on it became clear that I would spend my life helping animals. The question was, "How could I do that and get the best results?"

I was introduced to the concept of energy healing in 1986, when my little sister was diagnosed with brain cancer. At that time, I was twenty-four and she was twenty-one. I just *knew* that the core energy work I had been learning could help her in her illness, but other people didn't share my belief system. In fact, I was met with a wall of doubt and disbelief. My sister followed traditional medical modalities until the end of her life.

Just seven years later, I employed the few techniques I knew at the time to try to save my beloved soul-mate horse, Pet One, from the colic she experienced upon giving birth to Pony Boy. I lost her, and eventually I lost Pony Boy as well. I made many mistakes with nutrition and training between the two of them.

Taken together, those three losses were an epic PhD in loss, health, illness, behavior, stewardship, and nutrition. It was also the late 1980s and early 1990s, and during that time many of my friends died of AIDS. All of those losses were difficult, but they ultimately led me to become a kind of midwife of energy—whether the energy was coming

1

into or going out of this world. I made the discovery that whether a being is animal or human, love and intention can shift energy.

So my introduction to the world of energy healing was pretty harsh and often disheartening. In fact, I could have lost all faith. But while I had no evidence to confirm it, I believed in energy healing with as much faith as I had in a Source energy. And now, many, many healing sessions later, I believe that energy healing and God/Source/Unconditional Love are interchangeable. Energy healing can be a technique, a modality, a technology, a perceptual shift, a prescription, a bizarre hope, a seemingly endless cry, an idea, or even a moment of joy. It can also be done right on the very thread between life and death, and land you squarely back on the side of life.

Once I became an animal communicator, I set about to learn a million techniques and modalities, and my energy-healing toolbox has become wide and deep. But the biggest thing I've discovered from more than twenty years of animal communication, energy healing for animals with health challenges, and shifting animal behavior is that when I'm working I become a standing wave of energy, a balanced blend of vibrating frequencies. This enables me to be in a state of absolute calm and emotional leadership. As a standing wave of energy, I can hold a vision for the outcome that trumps any technique, technology, or modality anytime.

Now I grant you, that idea is not an easy sell, and it's hard for people to grasp. But I've seen it work again and again.

Energy healing for animals happens as a result of three things: love, intention, and managing your own energy. I have discovered that healing is an ongoing journey, one that includes the journey of healing the wounds of the soul. It is about leaving no stone unturned in the attempt to heal, to cure, to preserve life and vibrant health, and to understand the emotions that set certain unhelpful patterns in motion within a being's system.

At the end of life, when staying alive is not to be, healing is about the journey to the other side, which for the one who is leaving includes closure, peace, and acceptance. For the being who remains on planet Earth and has been the steward for the departed, the journey could mean anger, release, grief, and many other stages of experience.

An Animal Communicator's Life

In my first book, *Communication with All Life: Revelations of an Animal Communicator* (Hay House, 2007), I went into great detail about the loss of both Pet One and Pony Boy and how those deaths plunged me into the world of energy healing and animal communication. I never thought that world would open up before me in so many amazing ways, but open up it did!

A lot of people are curious about what my life as an animal communicator is like. For me, no two days are the same, and no two weeks are the same. My life seems to flow in cycles, but here's how it often goes.

Wake up. Meditate. Feed ten animals. You think I'm kidding? Nope: four cats, three dogs, and three horses. Work out—either hike with the dogs or jump rope, which always involves dancing with dogs and cats. Wild fun. I try to get a horseback ride in, and then I keep going for about ten hours straight.

I've been working on this book, of course, and in any given month I'll write articles, blog posts, and newsletters. So there is a lot of sitting, writing, and dogs wandering up and wondering when we're going to ditch all that stuff and go outside to play.

When I'm home, I'll probably spend a couple of days talking to animals on the phone (via telepathy) and a couple of days at other people's homes or barns, talking to one or several animals there. Both the phone and the in-person sessions can include energy healing.

I might do some teaching for a program I started called Communication with All Life University. I teach animal communication, energy healing for animals, and more, through teleseminars, webinars, and local classes. Then there's the quarterly three-day intensive animal communication workshop I do at my farm, in addition to other intensives.

I take my show on the road too, doing weekend workshops and speaking engagements, and for four years I've led dolphin trips and other wild animal trips around the world, combining animal communication and eco-travel.

All in all, it's a very full life, packed with animals, people, and . . . energy every which way!

Why I Wrote This Book

Let's imagine for a moment that you live in a beautiful apartment in a very hip part of an exciting city. You have a great job that you feel grateful for and a wonderful Jack Russell that you *live* to come home to.

And then the complaints from the neighbors start to roll in. Guess what? While you are at work, your beloved dog is barking all day long and driving people nuts. Now here come the inevitable threats about bringing this up in front of the condo board. All that racket is against the building's covenants, and you may get kicked out of your apartment unless you get rid of your baby.

At first, you may feel defensive about your dog and get mad at your neighbors. Then you might wonder if this really isn't a great life for a working dog (they are bred to be *ratters,* for crying out loud). But what if you picked up this book and read through the modalities and boned up (!) on ideas about other things you could do? Rather than deciding to try to find your animal friend a new home, you might commit even more deeply to the dog you love and create a far happier life for both of you. That's why I wrote this book: I want you to know about every available option to keep your animal in your life.

I also wrote this book for someone who, say, has a beloved cat in kidney failure and lives in a rural area where the nearest holistic vet is a three-hour drive away. Whether healing is simply about making her as comfortable as possible or there is still a spark left for you both to fight the good fight, I want you to have every available option too.

And I wrote this book for the person whose animals are healthy and happy—and could be healthier and happier! Even animals that are doing well can use a boost now and then, a little more support and a little more contact. And many of the healing modalities in this book are a lot of fun too. Why not look for opportunities for you and your animal companion to have more fun together?

What Energy Healing Can Do for Your Animals

I have seen energy healing work wonders in almost any situation you can think of. Energy healing can help or even reverse the symptoms of allergies, diabetes, cancer, aging, nerve challenges, insulin resistance, infections, and much, much more. I can't stress enough how valuable it is in achieving true healing. Energy healing can support the nervous, cardiovascular, immune, endocrine, and digestive systems, and of course the chakra and meridian systems. It's also wonderful for challenges including hip dysplasia, arthritis, and overcoming major injuries. Energy healing is excellent for enhancing post-surgical healing and especially when your animal is fighting for his or her life.

While energy healing addresses the physical demands of illnesses, injuries, or conditions, it also helps release any emotional baggage that comes with them. If the challenge is simply emotional, energy healing will help fast. After all, animals can't go to talk therapy to process their emotions. Okay, they *can* do talk therapy with a good animal communicator—but you still have to move that emotion up and out! Energy healing can do that and so much more.

Psychological barriers, such as being afraid to do something again after an injury—a horse that was injured during a jump or a dog that was in the car when you had an accident—can be addressed through energy healing. Grief can be supported through energy healing too.

While animals aren't spiritual in the same ways we are, they do sometimes "lose faith" in humans and act out in ways I consider to be symptomatic of a spiritual breakdown. It's as though they no longer trust in people, and then they don't even trust themselves. Energy healing can definitely assist in rebuilding lasting trust and love.

A Quick Tour through the Book

I've divided this book into two main sections: fundamentals and energy-healing modalities. In Part I you'll learn the basics. Chapter 1 covers what energy is, how it works, and how the energy of each member of your multispecies household creates a combined morphic resonance. You'll also take a brief look at the invisible energy systems of the physical body. Chapter 2 offers some examples of animals' natural energetic state in the wild and how this shows up in domesticated animals as well.

Chapter 3 is all about emotion—energy in motion—your animal friends' and your own. In chapter 4 I offer a few stories to illustrate animals' energetic lives, as well as a few stories from my practice of amazing healing.

Chapter 5 rounds out Part I and gives you an important foundation in the energetic systems you'll be working with when you do energy-healing work with your animals. We'll talk about chakras and some of the systems of Traditional Chinese Medicine.

Part II is all about the abundance of options you have to work energetically with your animals. While people sometimes think of energy healing as solely a very subtle process that works on a vibrational level, you will find that you can shift energy in almost unlimited ways, including what you feed your animals, how you touch them, and even how you talk about them. Chapter 6 explores bodywork techniques. Chapter 7 expands on this with more hands-on work. And in chapter 8 you'll learn some principles of nutrition and the basics of homeopathy.

Chapter 9 offers an array of vibrational medicine techniques, from essential oils to crystals to magnets. Chapter 10 adds to the list with one of my go-to treatments, the Scalar Wave, and several other techniques to explore.

In chapters 11 and 12, the emphasis is on you. You'll learn to shift your own thinking in ways that will affect your animals, you'll put systems in place that promote healing, and you'll learn energy-healing tools for yourself—the emotional leader of your pack.

Then it's time to get started with energy healing! Chapter 13 covers the prep work you need to do to set yourself up for a successful healing session. And finally, chapter 14 offers a giant "toolbox," containing a series of comprehensive "tool kits" for all of the most common issues I see in my practice. For each health issue you might face with your animal companion, you'll find a variety of healing methods that run the gamut from what to communicate to your animal to nutritional support to appropriate herbs and flower essences to use. This is practical advice I've seen work time and time again, and I want you to have it!

Now I'll close with a couple of things to note: First, you'll notice that the animals I concentrate on most in the book are dogs, cats, and horses. That's because these are the animals I've had the most experience with—and that I have at home! Also, when you use the suggestions I offer in this book, please make sure you also have a great trainer and holistic veterinarian on hand for support.

■ ■ ■

There is no end to the ways you can contribute to the health, happiness, and well-being of your animal companions by using energy healing. Are you ready to turn the page and begin? I can't wait for you to get started!

Part I

Fundamentals

■ ■ ■

I have packed this book with tons of information on a huge range of modalities and techniques that you can use to help your animals live healthy, happy lives. You'll find all of these in Part II of this book. Before we get there, though, you'll need to have some grounding in energy work. So here in Part I we'll look at the nature of energy itself, the energetic lives of animals, and the energetic systems you'll be working with when you do your healing sessions—everything you need to know to get you primed and ready to learn about specific energy-healing techniques.

1

Ground Work in Energetics

Until one has loved an animal,
a part of one's soul remains unawakened.
ANATOLE FRANCE

Energy Is

It's time to begin your adventure in energy healing for animals. Let's start with first things first: energy *is*. It doesn't begin, and it doesn't end. You can learn how to transform it and how to use it. It can gain velocity and momentum or drain and fizzle out. But it never goes away.

And *everything is made of energy*, including us and the animals we love.

If everything is energy, then we are all connected by and to that force. Our own energy system either adds to or depletes another's, and likewise, theirs affects ours. We are using, giving, emitting, submitting to, and creating even more energy *all the time*.

What does this energy connection mean for the animals in our lives? Actually, it means *everything*. Let's start with the animals in our homes because they are as susceptible as we are to changes in the surrounding energy systems. They are part of the universal exchange of energy, which means they contribute to our energy (and vice versa) by giving, taking, and transforming the energy around them and us.

Take the case of my client Jack and his beloved eight-year-old tabby cat, Murphy. Jack was always the emotional leader of his house and a strong, rock-solid type of guy. The other day he called me, and his voice just didn't sound the same. He decided to share some devastating personal information.

"Joan, my wife, moved out three weeks ago. It was a sudden thing, and I'm so depressed. But that's not really why I'm calling you. I'm calling because Murphy isn't eating. What's wrong with him? I just can't take another problem in my life right now."

This was a pretty easy one for me to figure out. When Jack's wife left, there was a major energy shift in the house, and it was affecting both man and cat. Murphy had obviously felt the shift, the sadness all around him, and now it was profoundly affecting his feline system, to the point where his appetite had dulled. (Stick with me here, and later in the book I'll explain how to shift the energy back to a good place for your pet, especially during times of trauma or upheaval, like a death, a divorce, or a grown child leaving for school.)

Animals Sense Energy

Human critical thinking has lessened our need to survive solely through instinct, and that's a huge advantage. But it has also eroded our ability to perceive subtle shifts in the energetic fields around us—we've gotten more used to thinking than sensing. An animal's survival, on the other hand, is based almost entirely on perceiving energetic shifts. Even the animals in our homes, pets though they may be, retain the primal fight-or-flight instinct. You might meet their every need, yet their instinct remains, even though it has been watered down to some degree through taming and breeding. By the way, that instinct comes on even stronger when you leave your animals to their own devices.

Animals in the wild—whether in a flock, a herd, a pride, or a pack—have a leader at the forefront of the group. The leader can be benevolent, and it doesn't have to be a titan of great strength. Sometimes it's simply the cleverest individual in the group. No matter who it is, though, all eyes and ears are on this leader. All sensibilities are feeling what the leader is feeling and thinking. And everyone has a "tentacle" into the entire group to get a sense of what happens next.

Since our animals are part of *our* group now, it's not surprising that they are easily affected by our thoughts and emotions and any energetic changes or trends in our homes. This includes the energy we bring back from work or of what might be happening in our personal relationships. It's true: you're not the *only* one who is anxious because that potential suitor didn't call. Your dog is also experiencing a level of anxiety because he's in tune with your shifting energy. He senses that something is not right with you and with the energy inside the home/world you share.

Understanding Vibration and Frequency

The easiest way to understand the energetic landscape you and your animals share is to remember that energy can be described as a *frequency,* a *vibration,* an *electromagnetic energy,* and even a *current* (like the flow of electricity). In this book I'll use all of these terms to describe energy.

Just as everything is energy, everything has a frequency, and all frequencies are broadcast into the world as wavelengths. A frequency can attract or repel, and the wavelength itself can also contain information.

Everything has a vibration—in fact, we live in a fully vibratory world. A vibration has this oscillation pattern of frequency or rhythm to it. Whether you consciously register it or not, you can feel the vibration of beauty and joy radiating from a field of tulips. Each individual tulip—its color, its stem, and the soil it's planted in—carries a different frequency, and when they're added together, they vibrate into beauty. A space, a stone, a piece of dirt, and a chair all have vibrations. Manufactured objects maintain a more sedentary vibration than live, dimensional forms of life, yet as you have probably felt yourself, a room can have "a vibe."

Here's a case in point: it's easy to feel a good vibe when you walk into a close friend's house and to feel a not-so-good one when you walk into that new grooming facility you thought you'd try—and walk right out with your dog. Was anything wrong in that facility? Yes and no. There might not have been anything obviously wrong that you could see, but if you felt a bad vibe, your flight instinct kicked in. (I bet your furry friend was way ahead of you in the let's-get-the-hell-out-of-here department!)

It follows that the walls of a room where a trauma was experienced will "hold" that trauma in their cells and membranes until someone purposefully, intentionally, and energetically changes the vibration. A church will hold the vibration of the prior service, even when it is empty. Even a decomposing body is vibrating. You can't stop the natural flow of the universe.

The fascinating part of this is that all living things have the ability to change their own vibration. A dog, for example, can change its vibration just by trotting over to the dinner bowl. Dogs will pick up their favorite toy and, as they walk around with it, gain the energy of security or a sense of pride. The dog oozes happier energy when it's carrying that toy. I know a large German shepherd who might look fierce to some people, but not to his family when they're at home and he's carrying around his stuffed cow toy. A cat may have a magical spot where it likes to sleep, transmuting the energy all around that spot. And horses perform better in spaces where the vibe is good.

As electromagnetic beings, we all have a field of energy around us called the aura. There are many complex explanations for this that I'll skip for now so that we can stay on track. For this moment, imagine that each animal, each blade of grass, each animate and even inanimate object has a luminous body that surrounds and interpenetrates it and emits its own characteristic radiation. That's what I mean by an aura.

Energy Transforms

It's well known that the various forms of energy in the world around us—including chemical, electrical, heat, light, mechanical, nuclear, wind, solar, steam, hydropower—can convert to different kinds of energy and power our world.

The energy systems in a physical body are similar. These include chemical, electrical, heat, and mechanical energies. Any living organism can be a microcosm of either *potential* or *kinetic* energy—and can be a source of power itself.

Energy in motion is *kinetic energy.* Energy in a stored state is *potential energy.* Potential energy from several sources can combine to create kinetic energy. Think of a common battery. Even after the juice is drained, the battery is still there in mass. At this point, it is potential energy. Once it is recharged by another source, it still has only potential, unrealized energy. Then put that battery into a flashlight casing, another piece of matter that holds only the prom-ise of energy. Now someone needs light, has an intention of getting light, flicks the switch that harnesses the potential and *voila!*—the flashlight is transformed into the energy of heat and light! Intention alone is the kinetic energy that actuates the light. *Intention and other energies are powerful together. It's as if intention becomes a power source of its own.* This is fundamental to understanding how to approach energy healing with your animals.

And Now a Word about Energy Healing and Frequencies

Many of my readers and most of my clients want to know about energy healing as it pertains to their animals. There is plenty of information about energy healing in this book, but for now let's go with just the basics. Energy healing, energy medicine, and vibrational medicine all share something in common: a *frequency* is involved, and that fre-quency is *the broadcasting of a wavelength, fine-tuned by intention.* Even if the wavelength is invisible, its effects are not.

Here's an example. A client's beloved thirteen-year-old Labrador retriever seemed down for the count after a seizure. The vet offered up medical options, but my client wanted to know about energy heal-ing for the dog. Right there in the dog hospital, we carefully worked through touch, gently bringing the dog back into her own body by helping her feel her own energy. Suddenly, a listless dog, who hadn't been eating, gulped down a burger and stood up. Now that's a visible result! The lab lived three more healthy years.

Energy medicine ranges from thought forms to prayer to touching with intention to good, clean foods that support vibrant energy. Energy healing can be about finding balance in your life and managing time among all the things that are important to you. It can be breath work to lift yourself out of old patterns that don't serve you. It can also be a complex series of thoughts and rituals that a practitioner employs on behalf of you and/or your animal. An aspect of energy work that continues to amaze me is that it can be done while a patient is present through hands-on contact, or when they're sitting across the room, or in a different location altogether (remote healing). I've worked with many clients who live halfway around the world. I never have the joy of meeting the animal we've healed together, but I can tell you from long experience that distance is not a barrier to healing.

Energy healing unites body, mind, emotions, and spirit. It involves fine-tuning the universal life force, the energy within each individual. Traditional Chinese Medicine refers to the universal life force energy as *chi*. Yoga tradition calls it *prana*. *Kundalini* is another name for this energy, which yoga tradition says is rooted and coiled at the base of the spine and is a powerful reserve of energy for one's true desire.

Spiritual Energy Healing

Spiritual healing is also a form of energy healing. In this form, it requires or elicits faith or belief. Spiritual prayers, mantras, and chants are petitions for help that invoke solace, strength, and repair—a combination of energy work plus intention. A prayer, mantra, or chant that has been invoked by many people through time taps into ancient technology, maintaining its vibration and carrying an energy of its own. And all of the people who repeat those words become connected and contribute to the energy and power of the words. You can use spiritual healing techniques with animals as well.

When it comes to healing, it doesn't matter what religion you believe in or what your spiritual orientation is. No matter where you are in the spectrum of faith and spirit, I believe healing is a collective art that takes place among the seeker/patient/client, the healer, and the Divine.

There is a Divine being, ideal, or agent in every discipline that works on behalf of spiritual energy. It is bigger than us individually, yet is part of us, with us, and of us. Spiritual energy, in fact, is the connector between physical matter and the electromagnetic field.

Spiritual healing calls forth Spirit, Source, Great Spirit, or the Holy Spirit to activate healing on behalf of a patient, seeker, or client. Archangels, angels, fairies, spirit guides, saints, Mohammed, the Virgin Mary, Jesus, God, and Allah can all be called upon for help in prayer or ritual. Christ Consciousness, Divinity Codes, One Mind, the Matrix, Reiki healing symbols, and Sacred Geometry also tap into ancient wisdom and technologies. In spiritual healing you can use the energy of a talisman, a crystal, a lucky rock, a statue, or a memorial, as they hold the vibration of the meaning that is attached to them. This gives them transformative and even magical qualities that I've witnessed time and time again.

Transformative Energies

There are myriad transformative energies we can access and work with, including breath, emotion, prayer, ritual, intention, inspiration, blessings, our own thoughts, and other people's thoughts about us. Being energy itself, a thought can form a *mass* of energy, and if we were to measure a thought by weight, we could describe it as either heavy or light.

The Eiffel Tower, ships sailing across the sea, cars, computers, and your home all share one thing: they began as someone's thought. Then, through intention, thought became form. Not only thoughts but also colors, aromas, essential oils, and flower essences all carry frequencies that can improve our physical health and our emotional well-being. They can be lifesavers during our bleakest times and a way to amp up our joy in the good times.

Before We Get to Your Dog, Cat, Horse, or Hamster . . . A Little Physics

Now I want to take a minute to talk to you about physics. If you took physics in high school, you might groan at the thought, but stick with

17

me for a minute. I'll boil down what I have to say about physics into a few easy-to-understand paragraphs. It helps to know this stuff when you're doing energy work with animals.

Physics is the natural science of observing energy and matter in space and time. Unlike sciences that organize knowledge that is clearly observable and measurable, physics embraces the concept of electromagnetic fields, forces that may be seen or unseen, philosophy, and natural science. Physics can even be a bridge into spirituality. The following are some fundamental concepts in physics.

A *particle* is a small object that has volume and mass. A *wave* is the transference of energy from one place to another with very little effort, meaning the particles involved in the transference may have hardly moved. A wave can also be perceived as a disturbance. Two equal waves meeting together create what's called a standing wave. A standing wave is always stronger than a chaotic wave pattern—any illness or naughty behavior in your animal companion is a chaos pattern.

To explain further, when we look at any animal illness or misbehavior, we are looking at a pattern of energy, and since illness and misbehavior are challenging, we could consider that pattern of energy chaos, or an incoherent field. We can influence this pattern with intention. This is because an intention is a wave of energy that will always be stronger than a chaotic pattern or an incoherent field. In fact, a wave of intention is capable of collapsing a chaos pattern.

Morphic Resonance and Your Multispecies Household

I must mention English-born biochemist Rupert Sheldrake, who wrote a book called *Dogs That Know When Their Owners Are Coming Home.* You may know him as the first scientist to "prove" that animals and humans share a telepathic bond. He also introduced the theory of the morphic field, a kind of organized database of information in the form of an electromagnetic field that contains the activity of living beings, acts, and even thoughts. Sheldrake expanded his theory to explore "morphic resonance," a collective pattern of "behavior" based on the pattern of a specific group's field. Each species has its own morphic resonance.

In a multispecies household, all of these combined fields of energy create a unique new field. Our households are giant vessels of morphic resonance!

In fact, when we speak of animals as mirrors of ourselves, it's morphic resonance we're describing. The morphic field we create with our animals has a pattern of its own that influences everything within it. It also has a memory, and its influence extends beyond time and space. It has a *like-attracts-like* pattern, which is to say that we draw energies to our morphic field that are similar to our own energies. And anything that doesn't jibe with our field feels "uncomfortable."

The morphic resonance of a household that has, say, a dog, a cat, and a human will draw into it other animals that are of like resonance. That's why some animals just slip right into a new household as if their familiarity has drawn them into the perfect situation. This was the case for my client Ben, who had a beloved standard poodle and found a stray pug on the street. The pug marched right up Ben's front steps, found a spot on the cold tile landing, and made himself at home. And the poodle accepted his new pal with ease. Soon Ben was wondering, *How did we ever live without that little pug?*

On the other hand, if a new animal in the household isn't a like-attracts-like energy match, there can be a lot of friction. There would need to be energy transformation on all levels in order for the new and "unlike" being to feel at home. Say your cat won't stop hissing at your new puppy. All is not lost. The friction doesn't have to be permanent—and I'll explain later in the book how to merge such energies.

You Set the Morphic Thermostat

Now you know some things about morphic fields and morphic resonance, and you know that the energetic beings in your home vibrate together to create a unique morphic field of resonance. The combination of your energies becomes a collective energy field with its own intelligence. One of the most important ideas to grasp as you learn to work energetically with your animals is this: you (as the human) are the *emotional leader* of your relationships and household. You set the energetic, or morphic, thermostat.

What you do with your own energy can have a huge influence on the overall field. Do you want to set your thermostat to anger and fear, or give that dial a good turn and set it on harmony? I know what you might be thinking: *Joan, I try for harmony. I swear I do. But I have lousy days too, times when I want to cry or scream. Am I supposed to suppress my emotions to make my dog happier?* The answer is absolutely not. But what you can do is walk it off or talk it out before you hang out with your animals. Process your pain in the privacy of your bedroom while they're in the living room. Yes—close the door and leave them on the other side of it. If you board your horse at a facility and you're going for a ride after work, vow to always leave your stuff at the entrance to the parking lot. Shake it off and *then* go see your horse, and you'll be able to set the thermostat for harmony.

My dog Olivia and my cat Alexandria went through a lot with me when I had some real emotional upheaval going on. My mother died. Then I got divorced. Like me, Olivia was very attached to my stepkids, and it was hard for her when all of a sudden they were gone. It was a rough period. We all grieved, and there was a point when our collective grief could have taken us all into depression. But then we moved to Seattle and started a farm, and everyone began to feel better.

Then we had another setback when Alexandria disappeared. After a while Olivia and I added another dog to the family, and then two years after the cat disappeared, I ended up adopting a cat that was pregnant. Suddenly we had a very full house. Olivia, half Border collie and a 100-percent Scorpio, had her paws full—with kittens.

Then my father died. As you can imagine as I unfold this story, it was a tragic time for me. Within five years, I had lost both my parents, gotten divorced, and lost my beloved cat, and my stepchildren had moved across the country. I was bereft, and the magnitude of it all was crushing at the time. To make matters even worse, I snapped a ligament in my neck, my shoulder dropped, and all I could do was lie on the couch and work on healing—and I'm usually the go-go-go type. But that couch (which, okay, is actually a dog bed) became a luxury for me. For the first time, I could actually indulge my fantasy of lying around reading magazines!

While I was pretty much immobile, I was able to observe that the whole sequence of events was a pattern and that I had the opportunity to truly, deeply process the huge amount of grief I felt. But Olivia was grieving too.

"This grief is mine," I told Olivia repeatedly. "You get to be the dog. I need you to be the dog now." Using visualization techniques similar to some you'll read about later, I frequently placed a little white bubble around Olivia and then a separate bubble around me as a way of separating our fields. We were soul mates and partners in the household yet also autonomous individual beings, who were capable of having separate emotions and different experiences. I did not need her to take on my stuff!

I relate this story to show that I understand life can be a rocky emotional road that sometimes feels overwhelming. Yet even in my grief, I knew I had to take on the role of emotional leader in my animal family, that it was up to me to guide the morphic resonance in my household and help us all create more harmony. And, yes, I say "*help* us create" because Olivia is second in command!

The Invisible Intelligence of Energy

Now, you may be saying, "Okay, Joan, what does any of this have to do with my dog, who is doing Thing X, Y, or Z that has me worried/ frustrated/crazy?" It has *a lot* to do with your four-legged friend. Let me explain why.

Let's say you just had one hell of a day. At work, your boss was off the hinges, and your sister called to pick a fight. Then at the grocery store the car wouldn't start. It finally came to life and you made it home, but you walked through that front door grinding your teeth because suddenly everything in the world has become majorly annoying, including those cute Girl Scouts at the store who chirped and giggled while pushing their famous carbs at you.

Now guess what? All those thoughts and feelings you brought through the door with you carry energy. The minute you and your animals share a space, you all have a shared experience—like it or not. Remember the Peanuts character Pig Pen, and the messy puffs of dirt and dust that swirled around him wherever he went? That is what your aura looks like now—and there may even be some shards of glass in there! Your arrival in the house is jarring, at best, to the morphic resonance of the household. Now all of a sudden, your dogs, cats, and even guppies are feeling the aftermath of your challenging state of affairs. They don't exactly know that you brought the mail in with you and discovered the electric bill doubled this month; they just feel your anger and anxiety. In other words, they feel your energy.

Clearly, what happens in your home life is not the only thing that impacts your household. You can bring home the slightest event from the outside world "in your pocket." You can bring home someone smiling at you on the street or the bad news in your mailbox. All of these events carry energy. Your mother calls long distance to rehash that argument from last Thanksgiving? You might think you don't care as you listen to her while doing ten thousand other things. But that conversation is still affecting your energy, and the energy you contribute to the house.

The field of energy that surrounds all things, including you when you're in a happy mood and you when you're in a funk, carries *invisible intelligence* that penetrates our auric fields and our lives, including members of our animal families.

And it's not just moods that carry invisible intelligence. A variety of toxins also carry it. This includes environmental toxins around the home, such as poisons in cleaning solutions, nasty ingredients in beauty products, and of course by-products and carcinogens in food. These are very strong energetic forces to reckon with that invade your space.

Thoughts and feelings can also carry toxic energy in the form of lingering memories and unforgiving moments, creating a noxious gas of emotions—something as simple as a thought you can't seem to shake from the narrow channels of your brain. Without labeling specific emotions as negative or positive, you can recognize that some emotions carry a higher frequency than others. If you stay connected to the lower-frequency emotions without finding and learning the lessons in them, eventually they can lower the immunity of your field of energy—and degrade your household's field of energy.

Any threat to our health that occurs in our bodies is introduced into our field of energy first. Any observable disturbance in our physiology has followed a long trail leading up to the disorder. All bodies are built with the intelligence to survive and thrive, yet illness and disease arise from somewhere. While we are born with certain DNA and genetic codes that can set us up for illnesses, the onset of disease is triggered by our energetic environment, both internal and external.

This is true of behavior as well. Unwanted actions on the part of our animal companions can be the result of their exposure to something as simple as a teeny particle of information—a memory, an unconscious thought, or a bad experience—or exposure to something toxic in the environment.

One of the most common things people call me about is that their dog has bitten someone or is even starting to behave aggressively toward people in general. The other day my phone rang, and a frantic client blurted out, "My dog has nipped four people! He didn't break the skin, but I'm worried. I don't want this to happen again!" I confirmed with this client that even though no one had been injured, this was not okay behavior, and we needed to act fast.

I'll discuss this specific behavior problem later in the book, but for now I want to point out that the energy in my client's home was contributing to this challenge. The dog had been known for nipping before she got him, and she hadn't done much in the way of training him. She was assertive with the dog while her husband was more like the dog's "litter mate," happy to roll on the floor and play, but always mysteriously somewhere else when the dog needed discipline. Added to this, the husband didn't want the dog confined in a kennel, or even the backyard, because he believed in "freedom." These owners were sending this dog a very mixed-up message. They had set their thermostat to "chaos."

Invisible Energy Systems of the Physical Body

When you do energy healing with your animals, you'll be working with a number of invisible energy systems.

Chakras

First, let me introduce you to the chakras. Chakras are seven wheel-shaped power centers that exist in our auric field while also penetrating our physical bodies at points along the spine, from the base of the spine to the crown of the head. The Hindu tradition not only named these centers but also attached an emotional perception to each. Each chakra also has a physical location and an associated organ, nerve center, and endocrine system gland, as well as its own theme.

Meridians

Meridians are an energetic map of the physical system with specific themes that illustrate or demonstrate for the practitioner or owner the true source of an energetic challenge, as well as ideas on how to heal it. Each of the meridians (with the exception of the Governing and Conception Vessel) is connected to an organ that has an emotional component. The meridians are also associated with and are influenced by yin and yang—complementary states. Yin is viewed as the female principle, passive, and more sedate, while yang is male, active or dominant.

When we think of a flowing river, the river has a life force of its own. It moves forward. When a big boulder falls into the water, this creates a disturbance in the river's pattern, and the water has to go around it. This is what an illness or injury is to the system. The meridians allow us to find that disturbance and follow it to its source, as well as giving us the ability to move the energy back into balance.

Neural Pathways

Another invisible energy system at work is the neural pathways we form in our brains. Every time we learn something and apply it, we create a neural pathway, and after doing the same thing a few times, that pathway becomes ingrained. It's why we don't need a manual to tie our shoes! Neural pathways are like well-trodden grassy paths, where the blades are bent over from repeated footfalls; it will take some time with no one on the path for the grass to recover. This is why, as NASA has proven, breaking subconscious patterns takes thirty to sixty days of brain training. The invisible path can be retrained to become a different route, or we can create a new path altogether.

When my father died, Olivia grieved with me, even though it wasn't really a loss for her, because our household had experienced so much loss by then that grief was a known neural pathway for us. It is easy to slip into known, familiar emotions and states of energy. The trick is to be the emotional leader and to easily and effortlessly guide your animals out of that state if it is not theirs to experience.

We're talking about neuroplasticity here. Today we understand that the brain is actually more mutable—more elastic or plastic—than we ever thought it was. We used to think that when the brain knew something, it knew it forever, and that it couldn't change. The brain was thought to remain *physically* the same. It turns out, however, that the brain has the ability to change and morph according to its experiences. Sensory pathways can actually bring about these shifts.

Here's what this means for us and our animals. It's not just because of the morphic resonance of the household that unwanted behavior seems set in stone. It starts with us because we are the "brains" behind it all. We have an expectation that the dog is going to dig in the yard forever or that the older cat is going to go after the younger cat. We focus on the activity and behavior we *don't* want and thereby set up a pathway for that image to play out before our very eyes. And then we're surprised when it happens again! But when we change the thought—leave that well-worn neural pathway and create a new one by thinking a new thought—this will change the energy and the behavior.

The same could be said for health and healing. If we have experienced loss over and over again, or if we've lost someone after a long illness, it can be hard to even hope for a return to health, let alone a miracle. The set point in our mind is that our animal friend's health will diminish, or even that death is imminent.

Nerves

Nerves are another invisible force we work with. Nerves follow pathways in the body and enable its parts to work. They also have their own memory. In the case of an injured leg, massaging and stroking

long the pathway of the original working nerves can
remember" their job and bring back the function of
important to remember this pathway with regard to
People are known to feel pain where a missing limb
used to be, so it would stand to reason that an animal would as well.
And sometimes animals lose parts of their bodies because of us: think
how many breed standards require modifications like shortening the
tails or clipping the ears.

Cellular Memory

Then there's cellular memory. Your cells hold the memory of your
genetic being, your DNA, and your mental, emotional, physical, and
spiritual being. Your cellular memory knows the patterns for illness as
well as wellness, and the cells can be informed to change, restructuring
the cellular memory.

Muscle Memory

Finally, we have muscle memory. On the positive side, muscle memory
is part of how we remember how to ride a bike or play the piano. A
practiced musician may recall an entire symphony within her fingers
as she listens to another orchestra perform it. Muscles also remember
trauma, as do the surrounding tissue, tendons, and ligaments. Muscle
memory can evoke fear and create "lameness" long after the pain, discomfort, or agony has passed.

■ ■ ■

All of these invisible forces come into play when we do energy healing
for animals.

How Does Energy Healing Work?

All right, so now you know a lot of things about energy and energy healing that are important to have in your back pocket as you read through
the rest of the book. But how exactly does energy healing work?

Energy healing can be described as making very subtle changes in the energy that makes up all things, including your animals. An energy-healing session doesn't always effect an instant "cure." It might offer a momentary respite, a different perspective, or a shift in some cells. Ultimately, as many individual cells shift together, they can create a change in the biology, pathology, or physiology of the animal.

Energy healing *can and will* affect behavior as well. It can be used to calm down even the most turned-inside-out beings, who have you at your wit's end, or to bring out a joyful personality from within the shell of an animal suffering from post-traumatic stress disorder.

One of the most beautiful things about energy healing for animals is that animals don't believe or disbelieve in any of the energetic technologies. When it works for them, it's because it's right for their being. If it doesn't effect a change, it's not the right fit. It is certainly one of the quickest ways to prove that these technologies can work since an animal's belief system doesn't stand in the way. Animals don't lie about how they feel, there's no such thing as a placebo effect for them, and many of the results of the energy work with them are specific and measurable.

While animals often respond to energy healing by getting better, it's important to understand that "healing" doesn't necessarily mean the animal is going to live. It can mean that they are going to more easily transcend into the next phase of their soul's journey. Thoughtful, intention-filled, directed energy healing can provide space, peace, and solace for the transition of all involved.

And Now for a Little History

You'll be working with your animals here in the twenty-first century, but before you dive in and learn more, I'd like you to know you're part of a tradition that stretches back millennia. It is said that energy medicine began more than six thousand years ago in China when the emperor, in failing health, needed the help of the local doctor. Problem was, the emperor didn't trust any strangers in the room with him, including the doctor, and so the doctor instructed the emperor's servant in what to do. He had the servant place needles in the invisible energy channels of the body called meridians. Then the servant attached very light threads to the needles, and the doctor adjusted them by feel while sitting in another room—with much success. Voila! The first acupuncture treatment!

Much later, but still a long time ago, the technique was used on animals. According to Cheryl Schwartz, DVM, in her book *Four Paws, Five Directions,* people were doing this as long as 3,500 years ago "when, legend has it, an elephant was treated for a stomach disorder similar to bloating."

Anointing the sick with oil is another venerable healing technique. It is a regular practice in many religions and may be the origin of aromatherapy. And then there's simple touch. The Bible refers to the laying on of hands as a way for people to receive Spirit, the Holy Spirit, or the Holy Ghost. The laying on of hands was also how clergy were instantly ordained. You received the touch, and now you walked with God. It was also a way of authorizing lay people as officers of a clerical establishment. For people of faith or those seeking faith, the laying on of hands brings great comfort, and comfort is indeed healing. Of course, the most famous hands-on healer in the Western world was Jesus.

Rule Number One: Start with Yourself

Okay. There's one more thing we need to cover before we close the first chapter, perhaps the most important thing to remember in energy healing for animals. Our ability to heal and help others *starts with our own field.* It is easy to project our own mental, emotional, physical, or spiritual challenges onto others. So, just as you're told to do on an airplane, you need to put that oxygen mask on yourself first and take a good, deep breath before you help others. Working with your own field is job one.

For example, as a practitioner, if I've woken up with a little bit of stiffness in my right ankle, and then every animal I connect with on that particular day has some sort of right hind ankle pain, I'm not doing my job. I've projected my own body onto the animal I'm communicating with, and that's not fair. A simple self-check is a great way to embark upon any energy healing or animal communication session. And I'll teach you how to do that before we're through.

■ ■ ■

Okay, now you have the basics under your belt, but we're not done looking at energy yet—not by a long shot. In the next chapter, we'll take a look at the energetic lives of some of our friends in the animal kingdom.

2

Energetic Life
in the Animal World

For the animal shall not be measured by man. In a world older and more complete than ours, they move finished and complete, gifted with extensions of the senses we have lost or never attained, living by voices we shall never hear. They are not brethren, they are not underlings; they are other nations caught with ourselves in the net of life and time, fellow prisoners of the splendor and travail of the earth.

HENRY BESTON

If you could swim to the right spot in the ocean, you would not only hear the clicks and high-pitched whistles of the dolphin community but also feel the web of their unique energy. The community of dolphins whose orbit you have entered, called a pod, exists as a unit. It doesn't matter if they are miles apart from one another or swimming playfully together, they're still a connected group, sharing a web of energy and a profound connection among the pod's individuals, family members, and the pod as a whole.

I have seen dolphin pods in action, and they're amazing to watch. They move together elegantly as a unit, as if choreographed, with full awareness of their surroundings and of all the individuals within the pod. If one dolphin becomes curious about something and drops back to check it out, the pod knows, and it will slow down and allow that individual to catch up. This is not just polite behavior; it's part of their flow. The pod appears to re-create its formation effortlessly, moving through the deep blue sea like poetry in motion.

These animals live in a harmonious vibration that is nearly undetectable to human senses. But what happens when the energy is not harmonious?

It's interesting to observe animals when they sense danger. Dolphins in danger swim more closely together. As for our animal friends on land, we've all seen the hair stand up on the back of a dog's neck. A cat's ears will turn to the side when it senses danger. A horse, at first, will not move forward. Then, suddenly, the same horse will turn on a dime and head off in the opposite direction at lightning speed. It's said that a horse can react five times faster than a human.

It's all about the creature's energy at work.

Watching Energy in Nature

A big ravens' nest came with the farm I inhabit, and a delightful family of ravens calls the place home. These birds have adopted me, along with my dogs, cats, and horses, as part of their bird family. I am honored to be part of their kin and often feel the protective nature of these animals. I see them fending off hawks that are about to invade our air space. They spy on my cats when they're out frolicking and warn me with their voices if coyotes are out prowling. What I love about the nest most of all is that offspring from years past make regular visits. They consider my farm a choice weekend getaway!

The large black birds always seem to shout "hello" when I walk past them on my way down to the barn. In fact, I've come to know the different calls of individual birds. If there is an eagle anywhere nearby, suddenly "our" farm becomes a no-fly zone. An eerie silence descends. Then I'll hear the eagle call, or I'll see her effortlessly glide away across the pasture. Score one for the ravens!

When spring rolls around and the ravens have their babies, I have a front-row seat for what I like to call Raven Flight School. The first time I witnessed it, I realized how clumsy baby birds are when they're learning how to use their wings. In fact, I can see it now in all birds—I had just never taken the time to notice before. But the first time I paid attention, I enjoyed the aerial demonstration from my deck, and I was able to tap into the energy of the whole circus.

If the babies took off across the field and didn't have their landing gear exactly right, I could feel the pressure on them when their parents screamed. When a baby landed on a branch—on purpose this time—bouncing up and down and shaking the whole thing, it screamed back, as if to say, "I did it, I did it, I did it!"

Like a showoff parent elegantly traversing a ski slope after their child has barely made it down alive, a raven parent will effortlessly sweep across the pasture. And so it goes, from tree to tree to tree through the forest. Raven Flight School is a very boisterous activity.

Beyond the physical reality of developing muscles and feathers, the individual birds are connected to each other on a deep level, through a web of energy, through telepathy and morphic resonance.

Speaking of which, a group of orcas or killer whales will work in unison to take down a humpback whale—an unpleasant notion, I know, but a reality of nature. Yet nobody in the pod shouts out orders. When an individual animal is on this mission, there is no time for signaling. It's as if everyone in the group has been handed "the memo," and they all do their part. It is beautiful, unspoken cooperation.

The truth is, an entire world of animal energy surrounds us at every single moment. As humans, we don't usually take the time to notice, so we miss the subtle cues, the differing squawks and squeals of the birds or the flick of a deer's ear. We also miss how animals function when they're truly tested.

Survival through the Senses

Animals survive by using the flight-or-fight mechanism inherent in their physical makeup. A part of the sympathetic nervous system, this response fires off the extra adrenalin needed to cope with danger. It's why a horse can run miles with a broken leg, or a mother bear can run into a forest fire to get her young. In our human world, it's how a mother can lift a car off of her child. Flight-or-fight bestows a nearly supernatural power. And it is based in the senses, not in language.

Language, consisting of words and rules for using them, is what we rely on to describe a concept, a series of feelings, or a movie perhaps. But language does not exist in the animal kingdom except insofar as we use our language to guide the animals in our lives. Animals have their own systems of communication: various vocalizations, body language, and many other, subtler forms.

Animals in the wild are dependent upon their senses for survival. Primates and elephants communicate by sensing the ground. Elephants respond to the seismic vibrations of the earth, listening through their limbs and reacting accordingly. Primates feel vibrations through their lips, hands, and feet. These lower vibrations, or frequencies, of the earth are associated with survival, and they are felt in the body.

Caitlin O'Connor has lived with elephants and written extensively about her findings, and she discovered that the elephant brain has a built-in backup plan of vibration for elephants in the herd who can't hear. Other studies indicate that a similar backup plan can kick in for some deaf humans as well.

Survival drives the vibratory connectedness between animals. Vibratory connectedness is what makes all the elephants of a herd take notice of another elephant's seeming misstep hundreds of miles away—the entire herd knows exactly what that means. It makes a flock of pigeons suddenly leap up from a phone line in the city, fly madly in apparent chaos, and land together on top of a building two blocks away. Nobody sees "the call of the wild" that prompted this, though we can plainly see the results.

Animals in the wild fight over resources and territory. They don't keep score. They don't fight over a belief, an ideal, or a religion. They don't strategize to take over the way humans do. Yet when animals work together for survival or a territorial takeover, in a split second, an action plan is revealed, and we can easily see that the individuals in the group are connected. Ultimately, we see their cooperation—cooperation that can exist only because individuals connect to that unity.

There is a place here on the farm where the vibration is magical, a teeny little area that I call the Faerie Garden. It's a place where I love to meditate, a small oasis of Pacific Northwest rain forest, with giant fern beds, tall trees, and a feeling of pure enchantment. This is exactly where the ravens decided to live. Smart ravens!

One day, I went to this spectacular place to mend a fence. For some reason, I didn't have any dogs or cats with me, which is very unusual since we usually act as a multispecies pod of morphic resonance. Before I even entered "the magic zone," I felt something different and stopped dead in my tracks. Through years of practice with my energy field, I have learned to pull my field completely into myself and act as though I'm invisible, and I did that immediately. I was simply a pair of eyes peering out of an invisible body. I even made my breath small.

Continuing to pull in my field, I concentrated on my breath. In and out. In and out.

Was the different vibe here in the zone some kind of threat? Was it a bear? A coyote? Maybe even a cougar? I concentrated solely on allowing my breath to be small and moved only my eyes. It was then that I looked into the frightened eyes of a three-month-old deer, frozen to the spot. I realized *I* was the threat I was sensing.

Continuing to take those small breaths, I moved my eyeballs in another direction and saw the terrified eyes of another three-month-old deer peering from behind a tree. To my other side, I discovered a third deer that seemed even younger.

They had been as attracted to that sacred space as I was, and I understood that. And now I knew what felt different about this place. It was *their* fear.

In that moment I knew exactly what I needed to do. I remained frozen as a statue and sent out the message, through vibration, "I am safe." I continued to make my breath small and my being just another random part of the landscape. Yet every exhalation sent out a wave of "I am safe." In no time, the baby deer started moving, released from their wariness.

By this time I felt as though I, Joan, did not exist. My body was a mere representation of the energy of a fun, playful, and loving being who was embracing these beautiful creatures. I was simply breath.

Then the deer's movement ramped up into play, and before I knew it, I was at the center of their running and bucking and leaping, feeling like a human maypole built for a baby deer dance. I could taste the energy of that playfulness—that's how big it was. In no time, fear energy had been trumped by deer joy!

This story takes me back to the dolphins I started this chapter with. When I swim with these special animals, my message is utterly clear: "I'm just here letting all of you know I love you." As I did with the deer, I shift my energy in that moment, and the next thing I know, thirty dolphins will want to play with me and the rest of the human pod surrounding me.

CONNECTED THROUGH THE BREATH

A little known fact about the connectivity of all life on the planet is that we all share the element of argon, a noble gas that is part of the atmosphere. Argon is present in our breath, in every in-breath and every out-breath. Souls, people, and civilizations come and go, yet argon continues. We could all be breathing the argon breathed by Jesus Christ, Annie Oakley, Rin Tin Tin, the cats of Egypt, and Secretariat, to name a few famous breathers that come to mind. In other words, we are all connected—literally, scientifically, and across time—through the breath.

Animal Superpowers

The magical and mystical ways of animals in the wild make it seem they have been bestowed with superpowers, but they are part of the animals' physical and energetic being. Sadly, these powers erode when domestication ensues.

The superpowers of the wild creatures include echolocation; protective eyelids; sonar; the ability to see energy fields, patterns, and grids; being able to jump six feet into the air from a standstill; and going from zero to sixty miles per hour in one minute, among many, many others.

Wild animals' eyes and ears work in ways different from ours—which helps explain why our domestic animals' reactions to things can seem extreme. It also explains why they appear to access a sixth sense.

Dolphins, a few whales, bats, shrews, and some nocturnal birds employ echolocation or sonar, sending out signals or sounds and listening for how they bounce back from various objects in the environment. They can detect safety, predator, and prey in this way. They have the ability to "see" without seeing and to communicate without language while being in a state of instinctual knowing. It's as if the eyes and ears are working as one and you can't really tell which sense is dominant.

Another supercool protective feature many species have is the nictitating membrane, what's also referred to as a third eyelid. This comes in handy if you are a peregrine falcon diving toward your prey from a mountaintop at two hundred miles an hour. If you're a polar bear, the third eyelid protects you from becoming snow-blind. Many other reptiles and birds have it too. It exists in dogs and cats but is tucked up pretty high and can only be seen when you gently open the eye and look for it.

It is believed that migrating birds and many other bird species can actually see the earth's magnetic field by means of molecules in their eyes or brains that respond to magnetism. They may simply be seeing the magnetic patterns of north and south, and this is what they follow. Salamanders and frogs also use a magnetic sense for orientation.

Our human superpower, on the other hand, is logic. We look both ways before crossing the street. If we get burned once by sitting too close to a fire, we tend not to sit that close again without a very good reason. If a dog is burned by embers from a fire, it won't go near fire again, unless we can talk the dog into it, reassuring it with a calm voice and our *energy*. I know if I work out in the morning, I'll feel better all day, so I work out. But a domesticated dog runs because it's fun in the moment.

Logic tells me that if I roll in deer poop, I will stink and need a bath. Yet one of my dogs always seems surprised when, seemingly out of nowhere, I want to put her in the bathtub. It doesn't occur to her that deer poop had anything to do with that spontaneous bath. In the dog's mind the thinking goes, *There's deer poop—awesome! What? Why a bath now? I smell so good!*

ARE ANIMALS COLOR-BLIND?

There's an old-school theory that animals are color-blind. True or false? It's true that scientists have found lesser degrees of color sight in animals. For example, horses have dichromatic vision: they see two wavelengths of light. Meanwhile, birds may actually see more colors than humans because their eyes have double cones in addition to rods.

Color holds vibration, and it may be true that more color gets translated to us and the animals through those vibrations than through rods and cones squeezed into that teeny optic nerve.

Many animals also have a tapetum lucidum, a layer on the back of the eye that acts like a mirror—that's why when you flash a light on them, it reflects back at you. The tapetum lucidum helps them see better at night, though it can also make them look pretty scary to us!

The Energy Signature

All forms of life have an energy signature, a frequency that is species specific. And within each species, individuals of all kinds—human and animal—carry their very own signature that is imprinted in their soul. The soul's expression as a particular individual is imprinted in the universe, and this imprint is then recorded in the Akashic Records. *Akashic* is a Sanskrit word that means space or ethers, so this means the imprint of the individual is recorded in the invisible web of consciousness. In heaven or the afterlife, an individual soul reviews this "recording" of its previous life.

Animals Make Contracts

Just as is true of humans, the soul of an animal being is a spark of the Divine. Some might call this spark the heart center, consciousness, or mind. Whatever you call it, the common thread is that the soul is the immortal "thing" that carries on when the body dies. The soul also carries the imprint of the past lives of a particular being as well as the setup for future lives. The soul contains the key to a being's journey and purpose and its "contract" with God, Source, the Divine, or the Universe. It is the connector between all beings. Regardless of the contract or the personality that is played out during each lifetime, the constant is the particular soul.

Also like humans, animals not only have a divine contract with their soul, they also share a unique contract with other beings. Humans have a different contract with a son or a daughter than they have with a life partner, and these are different from the contract between an employee and a boss. It is the collection of contracts between beings that facilitates each individual's playing out their karma. It's helpful to understand that a dog in your house will have a different contract with you than it has with your cat or your spouse.

For animals, again as with humans, karma is the law of cause and effect. A being's actions plant a seed that blooms over a lifetime. I don't think of karma as the saying "What goes around, comes around." That's just too simple. It isn't necessarily retroactive or dependent on time, because the blooming and the placement of a seed can happen simultaneously. Like contracts, karma is a very personal journey that an individual rarely fully realizes. It is about being causal in your own reality.

All life has a purpose, even if it is simply to be, grow, and thrive. Some life forms have a very obvious purpose. For example, we plant some flowers simply for their beauty and others for their medicinal qualities. Some life forms seem to have a built-in work ethic, with work as their purpose: ants never seem to sleep, for example, and bees are the archetype of busyness.

Yet an individual bee may also have the purpose of participating in your karma and a contract for deepening your intuition. Let's say you are out gardening, and you somehow know you'd better not go over to a certain section of your yard right then. A little voice says, "Quit gardening now; it will all be there later." But you don't listen to your intuition and instead power through and continue gardening, moving to that section of your yard. If a bee stings you there, you might say to yourself, *I knew I should have finished up and gotten that frosty cold iced tea instead. I need to start listening to my intuition more!*

One of the hardest things to accept is when our animal's contract is different from our hopes and dreams for our life with it. For instance, we might go to great lengths to help our animal recover from illness even though it may not be meant to be. When we approach energy healing, we have to be open to the idea that the healing work we are doing could be to make their transition easier.

One Mind, Swarm Behavior

Along with the individual soul, karma, and contracts, there is also the collective One Mind connection, invisible but always present everywhere, like the argon gas in the air.

Think of aspen trees. A grouping of aspens is really a single tree that shares a single root system; the individual trees are clones of one another. The group carries a central intelligence and frequency; one tree affects the whole collective.

Schools of fish appear to operate from a central intelligence, sticking together to defend against predators. When a school of fish decides to go in a new direction, it does so elegantly, moving through the water as though each fish is participating in a gloriously choreographed ballet. How do they do this as one? What we can see or measure is that they have eyes on the sides of their heads, the ability to take in stimuli around them, and pheromones they respond to in order to know what to do next. Yet they seem to also operate from a vibe that relays the vital information: *It's time to go this other way.*

This vibe that schools of fish, colonies of ants, and flocks of birds operate within has been given a fancy term: swarm behavior. Though they seem to be leaderless, these groups operate with an intelligence that leads their movements, a self-organized form of biology. Swarm behavior and morphic resonance have real similarities, as both appear to involve a shared energy field.

Swarm behavior is also evident in feral animals, which react to potential threats that are not perceptible to the human eye. Yet even one level of domestication will change the game a bit when it comes to how an animal will react. At the same time, there is that piece that is still wild. We see this in Bengal cats, mustangs, the offspring of feral cats, wolf hybrids, and certainly in many birds.

I get to witness swarm behavior on a daily basis at my house in my multispecies family unit. If I'm careless enough to leave food on the counter before I go out, the minute I walk back through the front door, the dogs try to swarm right out the door past me—the self-organized biology of avoiding a lecture. Even the cats look guilty. Everyone seems to participate in the "it-was-worth-getting-in-trouble-over" morphic resonance, even if it earns them an eye roll from the human.

Observing Energy in Domestic Animals

Sheepherding dogs are amazing to watch. Remember that these canines operate on a special vibratory level whether a human gives a command or not. Sheepherding dogs are so tuned in to the formation of the sheep and keeping them organized that a sheep could merely think about stepping out of bounds, and before it could take a stray step, the dog would be right there to put it back in line. It's as if these dogs are not only tuned in to their own task and person but also can penetrate the sheep energy signature!

Now let me take you into a barn in Los Angeles where I've enjoyed riding horses. I used to refer to this riding arena as "the spooky arena" because there was one place in it where the horses would always spook. It didn't matter which horse you took there; the first time it worked in that arena, every horse had the same startled reaction. And then, of course, we humans reinforced the spookiness by calling it the spooky arena. But there must have been something there that they could sense because, to a horse, they seemed convinced there was a boogey man lurking there.

I know dogs that refuse to go down a flight of stairs because that's where they fell once—as if the stairs themselves had caused the fall. Now stairs have a monstrous vibration for this dog. I knew a horse that had a stroke and fell down. When he awoke and struggled to get back up on his feet, the first person he saw was the groom. From that moment forward, the horse was afraid of that groom because he associated the groom with its being on the ground. It might sound ridiculous, but a client's labrador puppy was spooked by the sound of toast popping up. When I met him years later, the client told me that for the dog's entire life, each time a woman made toast in his presence, the dog would hightail it upstairs to hide.

As I mentioned earlier, the human superpower is logic. While we can't use logic to mitigate or change our animals' emotions, we can create energy around the situation or our own emotions. If an animal has a certain reaction to a person, place, or thing, we can tell the animal that the situation is fine, okay, and so on, but what we have to do to be effective is *show* the animal that *we* are fine and exude the calm that says "It's okay" in that situation. The animal will respond to this combination of persuasive communication and emotion—to that energy.

We can also take the charge out of a situation by purposefully changing the energy around it, finding something upbeat or fun to divert the animal's fear or panic, but we can't use our superpower directly. Even though we use logic to figure out that a specific diversion would be a good idea, our logic is completely meaningless to animals—they follow the playful energy.

Animals become overly reactive to things around them if the natural polarity of their energy field is skewed—that is, not aligned and in natural flow. Too much exposure to fluorescent lights, strong chemicals, and the electrical frequencies emitted from electronics in the home, such as TV and computers, among other things, can alter the polarity of all beings. In the long term, these environmental toxins can wreak havoc on health.

If they feel strange energy, an animal can become lethargic or the opposite, easily spooked. Their gut can also be off when animals feel strange energy. That feeling of knowing in the gut can set them off kilter, and then eventually the pH of their gut will actually change. Animals are just as susceptible as we humans, if not more so, to these intense things we have in our homes.

Animals also respond to certain energies of weakness. Some of them seem to have a sign on their back that says, "Kick me." I have known dogs that have repeatedly been attacked by other dogs at the dog park and horses that have been moved from home to home to home although each new person would say the horse had been abused for the last time, that this would be the horse's forever home—only to find that person would decide to move the horse yet again.

I met a horse, a true professional, that had been working at a cattle farm, just doing his job. When he was moved to a new home with my client, who happened to be a naturally gregarious person, a problem emerged. The horse of her dreams had recently passed away, but she was ready to love a new animal. Although Mr. Professional Horse wanted to please his new owner, he wasn't used to all the stroking and hugs my client had given her dream horse. So the professional horse shied away from her, and my client, who was devastated, began to compare horses. Her dream horse had been affectionate, but her new friend seemed cold and standoffish. Should she sell the new horse and try again?

I suggested that she pull back a bit, allow Mr. Professional to do his job, and wait for him to warm up. I could tell that this horse had no idea what to do with all that affection; he needed time to process this new type of energy. At the one-year mark, something suddenly clicked. Mr. Professional began to nudge my client and then went on to enjoy her strokes and hugs. In fact, the two became super close. They just needed time to size up each other's energy and adjust. I could tell there was a desire on both their ends to come together. It just took a while to get there.

I'm so glad my client didn't give up because now she says this horse is one of her favorite horses of all time. As he began to trust her energy, which he couldn't understand at first, this horse opened up to her and decided that life was not all about cattle herding, but also about a loving relationship with my client.

Think of it like dating. You might want a boyfriend or a girlfriend, but you can't pick somebody and glom on to the person right away. How would you feel if someone suddenly did that to you? So back off a bit when it comes to wrapping your arms around a new animal. You might be surprised at how your friend-to-be will relax into your energy and come to you when it's time.

Cats hold tenure in the university of teaching people great restraint with energy! We could learn a lot from them. When we come at an animal who doesn't know us with great excitement, it simply reads us as a ball of excited, nervous energy—and that can be hard to take! Think of how a cat incrementally makes up its own mind whether and when to sit near you.

We can have all the logic in the world that tells us, "Hey, we're going to do great things together!" But our superpower, logic, must be aligned with the right emotion for the time, and we need to exude the energy of safety and trust. We can't talk an animal into anything unless our logic is aligned with our emotional leadership.

■ ■ ■

In this chapter we got to glimpse some of the ways we see energy manifesting in the animal world, both in the wild and in our own home-sweet-multispecies-homes. But we're still not done talking about energy. Next we'll explore energy in motion, aka *emotion.*

3

Animal E-Motion:
Energy in Motion

When I talk about animals and emotions, I don't mean to anthropomorphize but to honor the emotions that are basic to animals and their similarities and differences from human emotions. We have all seen *National Geographic* images of an entire herd of elephants mourning the loss of one of its own: this is pure elephant emotion. Then there's human and animal interaction and the emotions involved there. We've all seen people dress up their dogs for this or that parade—St. Paddy's, Earth Day, Fourth of July—and we wonder, *Are we humanizing our animals too much?* (Mind you, this isn't something I judge. I've had a great time putting bling on my bemused cat, fantasizing an Arabian Knights costume for my horse and me, and watching my stepkids dress Olivia the dog in soccer shorts.)

Understanding animals' emotions has been critical to our evolution. For all humans, our emotional lives impact those around us—in the end we can all say, "Hey, I was here, and it mattered!" It's the same for animals. Even if that animal's life was brief, it still mattered. In the world of argon in our every breath and Akashic Records for animals too, all of our unique emotional lives—energy in motion—matter.

Think about a pair of eggs that burst forth, producing baby owls. Then an eagle swoops in, and sadly, those babies are gone forever. The mother owl's grief is a record that her babies existed, however short their little lives. The owl will carry on and breed again, and maybe next time, her offspring's lives won't be quite so short. Maybe one of them will live to be the oldest owl ever to live in that particular woodland. It's also true, though, that sometimes, just like humans, animals in the wild die of a broken heart.

This emotional imprinting also exists in our multispecies households, and it also matters. We each contribute to it as well as absorb it. Domestication creates a lingering emotional field and we mirror our emotions to one another.

■ ■ ■

A couple I once worked with, Jill and Dave, asked me over to talk to their aggressive dog, Annie, a boxer that had been attacking their adult daughter's dog. After a bitter divorce from an abusive husband, Maria had moved back into her parents' home with her pit bull, Buddy, so Maria could recover from the trauma. It's fair to say that the energy of the household was chaotic. Jill and Dave were struggling with the chaos of Maria's situation. They were resentful of Buddy's spoiled nature—and his doggy entitlement was not lost on Annie either.

Annie couldn't take the tension in the house and was taking it out on Buddy. It was evident to me right away that Buddy needed some boundaries he had long lacked, and that Annie needed some new forms of expression. It seemed she hadn't had a joyful, playful moment since Buddy moved in because Jill and Dave were so busy managing the situation that they weren't taking time to enjoy their dog. It took some time, but working together on communication and energy healing, we were able to bring the household back into the harmony Jill and Dave had enjoyed before Maria and Buddy entered the scene.

■ ■ ■

A thorough understanding of the depth to which animals feel holds the power to help us heal the emotional wounds they have suffered. It can stop the torture of animals in the name of science, and change the farming practices of the meat industry. Our ability to empathize with animals can help create more stable homes—for them and us.

Commitment to preventing their overpopulation can help us find creative ways to gather the resources to end the daily genocide in our shelters. Knowledge of animals' emotions can help create the focus on training that's required to ensure that no animal is left behind. And developing profound respect for animals' emotional lives can keep us from endangering the wild ones.

We forget that our superpower of logic holds no currency in the animal world. Yet it carries enormous currency in the overarching energy of the morphic resonance of combined species. An emotional leader can use the superpower of logic to create cooperation and trust with animals in the same way their pack, pride, or herd leaders would.

Animals will never make decisions in the same way we do, yet their thinking is remarkable and their emotions are palpable. They all exhibit their own species-specific superpowers.

EMOTIONAL LEADERSHIP

On behalf of our beloved planet Earth and empathetic caring for a multispecies world, we humans have to be emotional leaders, using our logic as a compassionate superpower, meeting other species' innate superpowers where they are, and combining all our emotions and energies to create and maintain harmony. We must never use our superpower of logic against the animals who share this planet. It will do no good. It holds no value in their world, and it manifests as cruelty. When misdirected, our combined logic and emotions equal trauma for the animals. In creating boundaries, we have to find a common language, which the language of logic is not, so that we can all understand.

Dr. Jaak Panksepp, a neuroscientist and the author of *Affective Neuroscience: The Foundations of Human and Animal Emotions,* has a theory based on the "blue-ribbon emotions" we share with animals. He writes that these shared core blue-ribbon emotional systems "generate well-organized behavior sequences that can be evoked by localized electrical stimulation of the brain."[1] In other words, you get the same behaviors when you stimulate the same areas over and over again.

These are the blue-ribbon emotions Dr. Panksepp says are shared by humans and animals:

- Seeking
- Fear
- Lust
- Play

- Rage
- Panic
- Care
- Grief

Cognitive ethologist and author Marc Bekoff writes, "Secondary emotions are more complex emotions, and they involve higher brain centers in the cerebral cortex. They could involve core emotions of fear and anger, or they could be more nuanced, involving things such as regret, longing, or jealousy. Secondary emotions are not automatic; they are processed in the brain and the individual thinks about them and considers what to do about them."[2]

I would add love, devotion, and embarrassment to the list. More on embarrassment a little farther on.

What Emotions Do You Share with Your Animals?

Imagine walking through the door and finding that telltale hangdog look of guilt or shame on your dog or cat's face. That the animals are feeling some form of guilt is obvious. We even see guilty behavior in horses—we know they know that we know. At the same time, it's as if our pets can't stop themselves from doing whatever it is that brings on the hangdog stance the next time they see us. Did they *like* chewing the rug or grabbing your socks and hiding them? Did they *enjoy* tipping over the open garbage can and playing in the mess? Yes, they did, and they're ready to apologize . . . until next time.

Bekoff believes we can learn everything we need to know about dog behavior by watching them play. There is a "wild justice," he maintains, because whenever their play gets over the top, they exchange apology and forgiveness—and then they go right back to play.

When I brought my third puppy, Delilah, into the mix of our household, ten-year-old Olivia reigned as the matriarch. Isabella, second in canine command, was Delilah's "babysitter," and the two would romp and play and play and romp until teeth were bared or snapped. Delilah would then go back to her corner for a while, but never for long. She'd always come running back to play.

Other scientists are evaluating Bekoff's studies because humans can learn a lot about fairness, cooperation, forgiveness, apology, and justice by watching dogs play.

As I mentioned, I would add embarrassment to the list of animal emotions. We've all seen a dog miss the ball, a cat fall off of a ledge, or a horse not quite make the jump, and next comes that sheepish look of theirs that seems to say, "Wow, that was painful. I really bungled that one."

Perhaps the most important thing for humans to note about dogs at play is that no matter what kinds of flare-ups occur, they're over in a flash, and then the dogs go right back to play. It's not that animals don't remember feelings and events; clearly, they do—and they may be a little more cautious in the immediate future. But their feelings and emotions don't linger. They don't hold on to them the way we humans do. We might obsess about how mad we were at our teenage daughter when she put a dent in the car while texting, worrying the thought like a dog with a rawhide toy. But the actual dogs? They go back to play. If we could learn that one trick alone from our canine friends, it would save a lot of marriages! We wouldn't place so much importance on past behaviors and mistakes, and we'd be better able to keep our emotional lives focused in the present.

Like embarrassment, the urge to seek is something animals share with us; the urge stems from our natural curiosity. This is why we check out the environment around us and connect with others. We seek these connections to enhance our lives. Humans and animals alike seek shelter and safety. We humans are no longer hunter-gatherers, seeking the fruits, seeds, and meats of the season, but we continue to seek food and clothing and other things that make our lives easier. We seek convenience. Diverging from the animals, we also seek abstract concepts such as enlightenment and wealth.

Humans and animals also share the anticipation of reward. We all have the capacity to look forward to something. For us, this could mean working toward a goal or counting down the days to major holidays we enjoy. Humans and animals are also similar when it comes to seeking attention, and there are common threads in how we seek rewards too. We might walk together after completing a chore or enjoy some playful grooming together after the day's work is done.

Like us, our animal friends seek basic needs, including safety, reassurance, security, food, and company. When we cover those bases, our animals purr and we humans sigh with relief. Different sounds, but both are expressions of contentment.

Then there are the not-so-great emotions we share with our animal companions, including rage. Rage in its pure, raw form is a result of feeling trapped. A milder form of rage is frustration. For you, this could be frustration from not being able to find your car keys after a half hour of searching. Your dog feels the same way when he can't find that bone he hid under the bed. Frustration also comes from boredom, the feeling you experience when there seems to be nothing to do and hours ahead of you with no stimulation. For animals such as horses, it's a very similar emotion; they get frustrated when they're stuck in a stall for endless hours and can't exercise. You go to work in the morning, leaving your dog with minimal access to potty and no real exercise or play, and when you get home, the neighbor tells you that your dog barked off and on all day. Your dog barks because he's frustrated. You'd bark too under such circumstances!

Frustration can also come from lacking a job or a sense of purpose. An animal in training can appear to be naughty when in truth they're simply expressing the frustration of not understanding what you want them to do. Take the case of a large German shepherd whose family just moved from a studio apartment into a big new house. He loves investigating all the rooms, nooks, and crannies. His job description—patrolling the house to make sure everyone is safe—has just quintupled, and he's thrilled. Many animals love to wake up to a task. Have you ever seen a dog fitted with saddlebags trotting back from the store with his human family? He knows he's doing something important for them.

And then there's another shared emotion: fear. Modern people don't react in the same way to fight-or-flight impulses as cavemen (and women) did, when life was filled with perils and they were always ready to leap into action with a weapon of some kind or flee quickly up a tree. But many animals still respond this way. Meanwhile, for us, fear can often be intellectual or concept-based. We can generate unnecessary fear with our thoughts, and that fear can sit in the human body and fester.

For animals, fear is very substantial. They react—fight or flight, straight up. In fact, they sometimes explode, running or snarling and biting. Fear isn't a passive feeling for them; they need to act. They can also quickly sense fear in a human being and feel very uncomfortable around that person. It's not that your cat hates Aunt Mary; it's simply that Aunt Mary is standoffish. Or your cat might hiss at your beloved auntie because she senses a fear vibe, and that vibe means danger lurking somewhere. Your friendly cat, beloved by almost everyone, knows that something just isn't right with this new person who just entered your multispecies morphic field.

I also need to mention the most extreme level of fear: panic. This shared feeling is about fear of the unknown and the sense that there is something to lose. Humans panic when they lose keys, jobs, or loved ones. We put a lot of energy into talking and thinking our way out of panic, even if some of that emotion lingers in our system. Animals deal with panic, which often shows up in the form of separation anxiety, in a different way. Your leaving the house might cause your dog to panic for a few moments, but he'll soon get back on his regular emotional track.

Physical and emotional pain often stimulate a panicky feeling in animals—they know when they're in trouble. Trouble could mean a threat to their life, or they could know they're in trouble because they just raided the counter and ate the entire cooked chicken you were about to serve. In the case of the chicken, well, there's a reason your dog is pacing nervously around the house: that's the I-can't-believe-I-ate-the-whole-thing form of panic.

We can't skip over another common trait in animals and humans—lust. There is no need for further explanation! I will just say that you have your crushes, and they have their crushes!

Care is a human trait and a maternal instinct. You find it in the soldier who stops everything to bottle-feed a lost kitten. Care is inherent in both genders, though it often shows up differently. When we think of human beings as hunters and gatherers, we can note that both of these activities are rooted in caring about the group and its survival. Animal mothers and fathers take care of their young and their pack as well. Male cats will express care by grooming everyone in the house, including the dog!

Play is something all species need. It produces joy and breathes life into work! You can't beat the endorphins created from play, and that's what causes pets and their people to find all kinds of ways to play—and to do it over and over again. Animals and humans share a similar structure and physiology in the brain known as "a reward center." Whenever we cooperate or are fair to one another, the reward center fires off, and then that behavior becomes automatic because it feels good. We love doing it, and we keep doing it.

Let me close by noting that animals, both wild and domesticated animals, experience grief, just as we do. While we humans react to grief in all kinds of different ways—sometimes expressing it, sometimes shutting down until we think we can handle the intensity of the feelings—animals are usually pretty authentic about their grief. Either they will keep moving, as is their nature, or they will show signs of their distress, which can manifest as listlessness, loss of appetite, sleeping a lot, or isolating and not engaging with others.

■ ■ ■

Pretty soon we'll start getting into the heart of energy healing for animals. In chapter 5 we'll begin with a more in-depth tour of the energetic systems of the body you'll be working with in your energy-healing practice. But not yet! First, I have a few more stories and ideas I'd like to share.

4

Animals and the Unseen Force of Energy: A Few True Stories

The animals of the world exist for their own reasons.
They were not made for humans any more than black people
were made for white, or women created for men.

ALICE WALKER

Our multispecies households are an ongoing experiment in energy. Whether we're bogged down energetically in an emotional state or simply having feelings about something, we can be sure that we *are* affecting our multispecies household. In fact, our animals may force us to become more conscious of this! Consider "the butterfly effect," the idea that a hurricane can form in one part of the world because of a series of events in another part of the world that started when a butterfly flapped its wings. It may seem like science fiction, but there is truth in it—the energy we generate can have impacts far beyond ourselves.

Morphic Resonance at a Distance

The other day I went to catch my horses in the pasture. They were all worked up, racing back and forth as a herd. What were they sensing? Their pasture mate Doc, a horse my friend Kelli owns, was not among them; he was off on a trail ride. Were they upset because Doc had been gone for too long? Had something from the woods set them off? Either way, it was plain that their harmony was way off, their energetic thermostat cranked up to panic mode. And this was very unusual.

I knew the exact time this was happening because my dressage trainer was about to show up, and I was afraid it would take forever to catch my horses and I'd be late. After the herd's panic ran its course and I caught my horses and tacked them up, we had a lovely lesson. The panicky energy was a forgotten thing of the past. Then my friend Kelli returned riding Doc, and I told her what happened.

"What time was this?" she asked me.

"It was one o'clock, on the dot."

"Well that's funny, because right at one Doc was starting to spook, to the point where I started wondering if the safest thing to do would be to get off him. But then he calmed down."

"When did he finally settle?" I asked Kelli.

"About ten minutes later, I'd say."

That was the same amount of time it had taken for my horses to settle.

At the time the herd got worked up, Kelli and Doc were more than three miles away, yet the horses' morphic field spanned that distance. It was the butterfly effect, or swarm theory, in full operation!

Emotional Leadership

I talked about emotional leadership earlier, but I can't emphasize it too much. The first step in supporting your animals energetically is to get some practice setting the emotional thermostat in your multispecies world.

With cats, you might want to do this for the sake of your furniture! Cats can pick up the displaced emotions in a household on so many levels. When those emotions are chaotic, they don't feel safe—and you'll know it soon enough, maybe in the form of a shredded armrest.

If you walk into a horse's stall feeling fear, depending on the horse, you could be met with either defensiveness or kindness. Horses can smell the energy of fear; they can taste fear. That's why when you're introduced to a new horse, you need to enter its space with the energy of confidence, respect, and compassion. Any animal that's reacting to fear has a keen awareness of its surroundings, and whatever the human in the picture is feeling will only magnify this intense awareness.

When I communicate with horses, they frequently tell me that a person in their life has brought all the baggage of their nine-to-five job—the worries, frustrations, or even joyful excitement—to the barn. Whatever emotional state their person is in, they can sense that the human isn't fully present, and this can be a real challenge for the horse, who is looking for emotional leadership. If the rider on its back is stuck in a mental argument with her boss, the horse has no incentive to play along with that energy.

Energy can build up in undesirable ways. Let's say, for example, a horse is in the ICU with a fever, and tests are inconclusive. The veterinarians are baffled, and the horse's people are feeling sad, confused, and helpless. This can create a snowball effect, building more fear, grief, and a premature sense of loss, and energy like that can work against the horse in its attempt to heal. As the emotional leader, you need to do whatever you can to find neutral again. You'll find lots of suggestions for ways to do this farther along in the book.

So energy begets more energy. Energy builds on itself. This can work to everyone's advantage too. A good example is what happens during training when the animal "gets it," finally understands what you're asking of it. You can frequently see *and* feel the light bulb go on for the animal, and the energy of that breakthrough and the resulting praise carry forward into future sessions. The emotional reward creates the desire to continue to do well, and when that happens, training is something they can easily understand—and it becomes fun.

The Energy of the Professional Animal

In competition, some animals have a certain air of professionalism. They are used to winning, have neural pathways carved out for it—no ifs, ands, or buts about it. I love watching the best-in-show segment of the Westminster Dog Show. I'll never forget an Australian shepherd named Beyoncé, who was just fantastic in demeanor and gorgeous to boot. Oh, but wait! The next dog that came out strutting his stuff was a phenomenal Tibetan terrier. And then came a long-haired dachshund who was equally fabulous. And on and on it went. These dogs had beauty, swagger, and grace. They were great examples of the breed standard—and personality!

I couldn't imagine what the judges would do because every one of these dogs deserved a ribbon. In the end, they picked a boxer, a beautiful, leggy girl with a kind face. And guess what? That boxer had won fifty-six best-in-shows by then. Her muscle memory, neural pathways, aura, morphic resonance, and soul's journey clearly, undeniably exuded *winner*.

In a similar example of winning energy, I once watched the jockeys mount their horses for the annual Kentucky Derby while the sports commentator bantered with Gary Stevens, a three-time Kentucky Derby winner. As the horses were being led to the starting gate, the commentator said, "Oh, these guys must be so nervous at this point."

"Oh, no. Not now. Now they have a peaceful calm," said Stevens. "They only have to trust their connection with the horse now. The work of the trainers and everyone else is done. It's just them and their horse."

Some animals carry a healing energy vibration. Therapy animals have a certain aura that exudes peace or inspires learning. The pure entertainers among them seem to know just how to make everyone laugh. Animals that assist humans in these ways are aware that their bright vibrations can shift the human energy field.

Bypassing Logic, Leaping into Faith: True Stories of Animal Healing

When it comes to healing, sometimes we have to bypass our own superpower of logic and take a leap of faith. I have seen many situations where a human working diligently on an energy technique gets results that veterinary medicine just can't explain.

Faith—trust in and devotion to something in our world—becomes its own superpower that can move us light years ahead of what we can accomplish going through the motions of logic. Whether we devotedly pray for miracles or trust in some sort of healing modality, faith takes us out of our heads and its concerns about past and future and instead puts us in present time. When we are present, we make the space for grace and miracles to happen.

Martin was a kitten with a congenital heart condition that usually showed up in purebred cats at about the age of four. But Martin was much younger when this condition appeared, and it was quite advanced. He was hospitalized in the ICU, and that was where his owner, Gloria, and I worked with the Scalar Wave (a technique I'll describe in chapter 10). His heart rate and breathing were being monitored hourly, and the charts clearly showed a dramatic shift taking place at the exact hour when we did our energy work with him (see the chart below). Martin was able to go home that week, and though he eventually did cross over, he lived a couple of months longer than any veterinarian had expected. And he died peacefully playing.

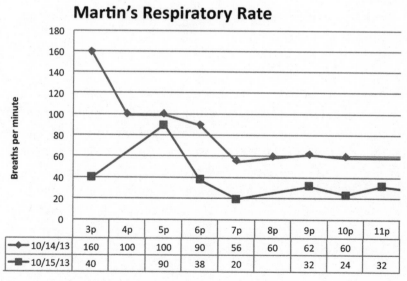

Martin's Respiratory Rate

	3p	4p	5p	6p	7p	8p	9p	10p	11p
◆ 10/14/13	160	100	100	90	56	60	62	60	
■ 10/15/13	40		90	38	20		32	24	32

FIGURE 1 The spike in the graph indicates how high Martin's heart rate was and how challenged his breathing was. We worked on him energetically/remotely at 6:00 p.m. and you can see the calming effect it had on both his heart rate and breathing.

My client Jen, whose dog had kidney disease, was able to measure his blood urea nitrogen (BUN) level before and after I worked on him using the Scalar Wave. This animal too was able to stay on the planet with Jen longer than expected—this time a couple of *years* longer.

Mangia was a high-level dressage horse that had been in training preparing for a competition. One morning she woke up with zero circulation in one of her legs. She was lying down when they found her, and it took everything they could think of to get her up. The veterinarians, whom the owner, Cindy, had called in from the University of Missouri, told her they were sorry that her horse would probably have to be euthanized. But Cindy wasn't about to give up so easily. She called me and asked for my help.

Meanwhile, I was in Florida, heading to the Bahamas for my annual animal communication dolphin trip. I had no way to do much more than a few remote rounds of the Scalar Wave technique. And I would be going out to sea shortly, without any way to find out what happened. When I returned to shore six days later, I was thrilled to find out that Mangia was not only still with us, but doing well. The vets were stumped by her recovery. But Mangia didn't care. She went on to compete the following spring.

■ ▪ ■ ▪

I offer these stories as just a few examples of what's possible when you take that leap of faith and help your animals heal by shifting their energy. I'm here to tell you that it works—I've seen it work thousands of times—and that *you* can do it! And now it's time to start learning how. You'll begin by getting acquainted with the invisible but oh-so-powerful energetic systems in your animal companions' bodies.

5

Energetic Systems in You and Your Animals: An Overview

May all that has life be delivered from suffering.

GAUTAMA BUDDHA

Much Ado About Chakras

You may have already heard of the chakras as an energy system that humans have. Animals have them too. To visualize what they look like, you can picture spinning wheels or discs, centered in the physical body along the spine and extending outward from the body too. Some see a chakra as a vortex, a whirling, three-dimensional mass. Perhaps it's easiest to imagine a cone-shaped funnel extending from the physical body, with the slimmest point actually planted in the body.

The chakras are associated with locations in the physical body and with themes. Think of it this way: each chakra, in either you or your animal, holds specific information based on individual history, and it also contains the potential of what each chakra represents.

Chakras are associated with colors as well. Here is a summary of the themes and colors of the seven main chakras:

- First: survival; red
- Second: power; orange

- Third: self-esteem or self-worth; yellow
- Fourth: the heart or unconditional love; green (although in animals, the color associated with unconditional love is pink)
- Fifth: creative expression; blue
- Sixth: intuition; purple, violet, or indigo
- Seventh: connection to God/Spirit/Source/Universe; white

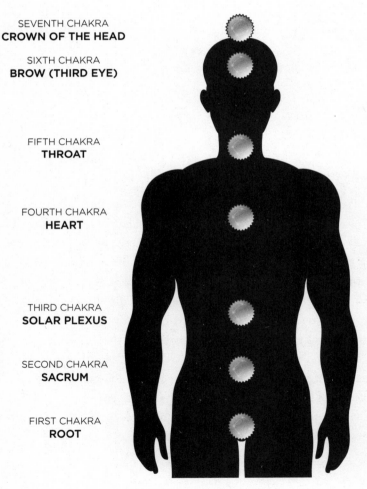

SEVENTH CHAKRA
CROWN OF THE HEAD

SIXTH CHAKRA
BROW (THIRD EYE)

FIFTH CHAKRA
THROAT

FOURTH CHAKRA
HEART

THIRD CHAKRA
SOLAR PLEXUS

SECOND CHAKRA
SACRUM

FIRST CHAKRA
ROOT

FIGURE 2 Human chakras

Imagine that the chakras categorize our experiences for us throughout the body. If something isn't jelling in our personal, emotional, or physical environment, these power centers can potentially lose strength, leading to illness. There are also behavioral repercussions associated with weak chakras. I always think of the chakras as different theme parks that are all interrelated—it's sort of like going to Orlando!

Through conscious thought and clearing techniques, each chakra also holds the potential to create wellness or better behavior. In the descriptions of the chakras that follow, I'll first focus on the human chakras—because, after all, your first job as the emotional leader is to balance your own energy—and then I'll move to an in-depth examination of animals and what a disturbance in each of these areas could mean.

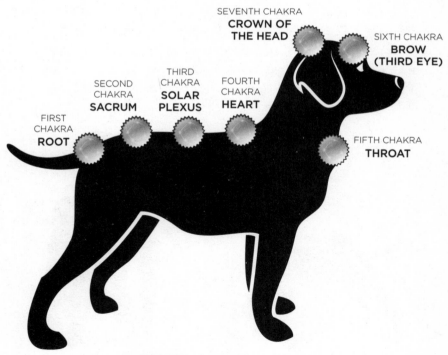

FIGURE 3 An animal's chakras

The First Chakra: Survival

For Humans

The first chakra is under our *sitz bone;* basically, we sit on this chakra. It is located at the base of the spine, the origin of kundalini energy. Kundalini energy is said to be female and lying coiled like a serpent, waiting to spring up the spine. Another term for kundalini is life force, so the first chakra is the seat of the ever-emerging and expanding life force.

The first chakra governs the immune system, the legs, feet, blood, bones, joints, and even the skin. This is also the home of our sexual organs and of male hormones. The first chakra rules reproduction; it is the seat of the drive to procreate.

The color associated with this chakra is a vibrant red. The first chakra represents the tribe and family: the family of origin as well as the family we have created to provide safety. It represents our culture, our country of origin, and our companions, friends, organizations, and work-mates. It is our home and our safety. It's also home to the life force. The first chakra colors how we view other groups because it represents emotional security and our need for safety. It holds the fight-or-flight instinct. It also represents being grounded on planet Earth and making sound decisions that embody our whole being.

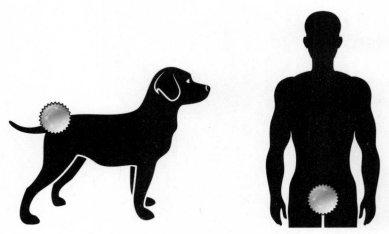

FIGURE 4   First chakra—color, red

For Animals

The first chakra sits at the base of an animal's tail—at the end of the spine. As in humans, the first chakra is also where the life force sits in animals. In fact, it is the driving force, literally, in the fight-or-flight response in many species.

Physically, the first chakra governs the immune system, the hind legs, and the hind feet. It is also home to the sexual organs—this time in females. It carries the energy for blood, bones, skin, and joints. In Chinese medicine, many meridians end or begin at the feet, and a combination of several of these points make up the *jing points*—points that enhance the immune system when stimulated as well as the circulation in each of the limbs.

As with our own chakra system, the first chakra represents security and safety for animals too. And as I've mentioned, they live in their fight-or-flight senses; these senses are always charged up and ready to activate. The first chakra also represents how grounded an animal is and how well they listen to a partner or a leader.

Finally, the first chakra represents the pack, herd, pride, flock, and even the multispecies pack that we create in our own homes, our multispecies morphic resonance.

TAILS AND CHAKRAS

Tails are outstanding communicators! As a cat walks through a room, its tail is a gauge of its safety and comfort. If it is straight up, all is good with the world—it's as though the cat is hoisting a flag of pride. A cat's tail at mid-level is a sign that the cat is checking things out. And of course, if need be, it can lower its tail to the ground and become like a hovercraft, scooting from point A to point B with its tail barely skimming the surface. That is not a happy cat, however; it's a cat in distress mode. And if a cat is angry, its tail will flick back and forth.

A dog's tail, of course, also tells a tale. Every morning before I even open my eyes, just as I'm coming to awareness, my dog Olivia wags her tail with feverish delight because we get to start another day together. She also wags her tail with joy when someone else in the household is getting in trouble—that's just Olivia!

A dog that's excited will wag its tail, and then its reaction can go in any direction. Whatever happens next, we know there is a high level of stimulation. Some people are surprised to see a dog act aggressively while its tail is wagging, but a wag is not always a happy wag—the tail operates solely from instinct. The excitement reflected in the wag can go to nervousness and fear as quickly as it can go to sudden "big fun."

What do we see in a scared dog's tail? We often find it tucked. Several studies suggest that a dog's tail wagging to the right shows a friendly feeling, while a tail wagging to the left shows caution.

With a horse, the tail indicates engagement when riding, while a tail that is not engaged usually indicates some sort of prior back injury. A horse will be very protective of this area. You see happy tails on horses, swishing with a staccato rhythm, and you see tails that act like arms to swat someone or something away. Physical signs like these can represent a feeling of extreme safety or fear.

The engine behind any equine discipline or canine sport is the hind end. The true locomotive for fight or flight is the hind end. It's interesting that most animals have some sort of greeting ritual around the butt, checking out the hind end. If the animal being checked out doesn't trust the situation, it can literally "turn tail" and leave.

Linda Tellington-Jones, an internationally acclaimed authority on animal behavior, training, and healing, has a theory that many aggressive dogs are very tight back in the haunches and that TTouch (her branded method of massage) can unlock this tension. Nearly 95 percent of the time, aggression in animals stems from fear or a need for protection, but aggression can also be the result of an emotional or a physical trauma.

Bodywork in the first chakra area is very good for enhancing feelings of safety in your animals. It is also good for relieving aches and pains as they get older. This area is tighter in the alpha of any herd, pack, or pride, because the alphas are more on guard. You'll also find more tension in a newly adopted or a shy dog. This is a good place to massage them to gain trust.

You may be surprised to find that first chakra massage works with a wide variety of animal friends. Years ago I had the honor of working energetically on a beautiful exotic rooster who had survived a raccoon attack and the sad loss of several of his hens. He felt threatened yet was the head of his flock. We worked primarily on his first chakra to restore his sense of safety.

The Second Chakra: Power

For Humans
The second chakra is located between the belly button and the pubic bone. Physically, it governs all of our reproductive organs, the bladder, hips, lower vertebrae, lower intestine, and the pelvic shield for all of these organs. It contains the female organs and hormonal glands. In Traditional Chinese Medicine, the bladder is related to shock. It's also the process center for elimination.

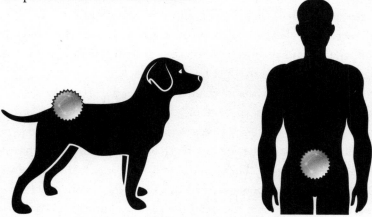

FIGURE 5   Second chakra—color, orange

Emotionally, the second chakra governs money, personal power, and sex, and it's about the feelings that come with money and sex: guilt, control, and the need for power. This is also the area that blames, and so it contains the energy of those we want to hold accountable. The second chakra is also about fertility and is where the spark of creativity is born.

The second chakra relates to how we see ourselves—and the view isn't always pretty. Frequently, we bury secrets here, which are later revealed in illness or sexual or hormonal dysfunction. The second chakra also represents our one-on-one relationships.

For Animals

To find the second chakra on animals, we look on the top of the animal in the region of the lower back, hips, and sacrum. This is the area that is visible, available, and vulnerable to the world.

As with humans, the second chakra governs the hips, reproductive organs, sacrum, lower vertebrae, and lower intestine. This chakra also includes teats and the male sexual organs.

The second chakra of animals represents sex, power, and their one-on-one relationships with other animals in the home, barn, or field as well as with their humans. Of course, this is also the power center for the human-animal connection. The second chakra represents other human power struggles that might affect animals, including money struggles, especially if they directly impact the relationship.

If any chakra takes on the mental, emotional, and physical human story, including our shadow emotions like guilt and shame, this is the chakra where an animal may get hooked.

An overactive lifestyle can result in a breakdown in the second chakra, an earned soreness. Certainly a racehorse that has pounded the track for several owners has earned the right to be a little sore here by the time it retires at the age of twenty-one. Dogs who have chased the kids around the neighborhood in family fun, watched their wards run off to college, and now get to lie quietly in the family room have earned their soreness here too. And the cat that jumped out of trees like Tarzan gets stiff here as well.

More and more, dogs and cats that are not spayed and neutered and are not in a breeding program are coming up with breast cancer and prostate cancer, diseases in areas governed by the second chakra. In busy spay and neuter clinics, dogs and cats can have their legs placed at extreme angles for extended times, often before the ligaments have fully developed in those areas, and sometimes permanent soft tissue damage results. The more animals in the lineup that day, the more likely your darling will remain in that position.

The result of being left in these extreme positions becomes more evident as the animals age. A dog might paw and paw and not quite be able to comfortably lie down because it's hard for its hips to get comfortable. I'd like to pose a question. What if we're seeing so much second chakra breakdown because we are taking our animals' procreative power away? Now, I believe in spaying and neutering; I'm not suggesting that we don't do these. But what if we did this more consciously? One way to do so is to go to a veterinarian you know and trust instead of a high-volume spay and neuter facility. It might cost a little more in the short term, but in the long term it will result in a healthier physical body and second chakra.

Since the second chakra holds the energy of one-on-one relationships, some of the questions to ask about this area include the following:

- How many households has this animal been in?
- How many jobs has this animal had?
- How much armor is this animal wearing to prevent more heartbreak because it has switched homes so many times?
- How many other animals have joined the household?
- How many people have come and gone?
- How much of our sadness and attachment to emotions about losses do we carry (and thus project onto our animals) in the household?

The second chakra is an excellent area to stimulate with massage when you are just lying on the couch with your dog or cat. As animals age and you notice weakness in their hind end when they get up, that stiffness usually starts in the second chakra. Keeping it stimulated with touch will increase the circulation.

The Third Chakra: Self-Esteem and Self-Worth

For Humans

The third chakra sits at the solar plexus and governs our stomach, liver, kidney, pancreas, spleen, adrenals, digestion, filtering organs, and glands. Well-known holistic physician Dr. Andrew Weil considers the stomach "the second brain."

"Itis" diseases in the gut start here as a result of too much acidity. Arthritis, colitis, and "leaky gut syndrome" are also related to autoimmune disorders. Adrenal exhaustion is a third chakra challenge, as are ulcers and diabetes (losing "the sweetness in life"). This part of our physical body operates as a filter via the digestive system, as well as the emotional system.

Emotionally, the third chakra governs self-esteem, gut instincts, and gut reactions. This area tells us whether we trust something or not. The third chakra is the lens that determines how we feel and see the world and how the world feels and sees us. This is the center of

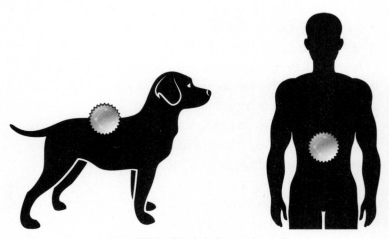

FIGURE 6   Third chakra—color, yellow

courage, get-up-and-go, and will. It is a true processing center, whether it works on food or emotions.

In Traditional Chinese Medicine, the liver is associated with anger, the gallbladder with frustration, the kidneys with fear, the spleen with worry, and the stomach with pensiveness.

For Animals

Animals enjoy the same third chakra gifts and suffer the same quandaries as humans. Although domestication has dulled our animals' gut instincts, they retain the fight-or-flight instinct, which sparks in the stomach.

Animals also have a twenty-four-hour weather channel in their guts. They can feel barometric pressure change hours before the weather actually changes, and this affects their behavior. We could have that sense too if we dialed into our own stomachs, but most of us have walled off the gut to such an extent that we aren't even aware we have digestive issues. Yet a dog that is affected by thunder and lightning can sometimes feel them approaching eight hours before they first strike.

Food and nutrition are some of the most important tools we have to support animal health. Many animals are afflicted by terrible human diseases that can be traced to digestion. Household animal companions and horses have food allergies, insulin resistance, ulcers, liver disease, and kidney disease, to name a few. Wasn't it bad enough when cancer in animals started to rise? Now we have replicated nearly every possible human disease in our animals because of poor food choices we are making for them.

Though more and more people are aware of what is in some pet food, they continue to make the same dangerous nutrition choice day in and day out. Pet food manufacturers use corn and wheat as fillers. When did a dog in the wild ever say, "Please, I'd like some wheat before the meat?" Does a cat in the wild stop off for some corn before carrying on with the hunt?

I teach an animal feed-label reading class. The first five ingredients tell the tale. It is amazing what passes for food in these "foods." When I pass out labels in my class and ask people to try to identify the actual food in the "food," they're often stumped.

All the internal organs associated with the third chakra suffer the consequences of how we feed animals. Trouble with the pancreas results in diabetes. The liver or gallbladder can reflect the anger and frustration of a household, which our animal friends stuff down. This plays out dramatically for them in their "unspeaking" world. Sadly, we pay for these third chakra problems in the form of vet bills and at the cost of losing them much too early.

The third chakra in an animal also involves self-esteem. Many horses have saddle issues in that area, and many dogs sag in this area as they age. Cats end up with kidney disease. Here are some scenarios that could lead to a breakdown in the third chakra:

- A horse that has changed jobs several times
- The family dog that has watched the kids it helped raise go off to college
- An animal that has been in several homes
- Animals that are picked on by other animals
- Animals that were not treated kindly in human households and are now scarred by insecurities
- The stoic animal that won't let on it is in greater pain than it lets on

This list represents just a few of the common issues that might drive a breakdown in this area.

Things that could quickly support an animal challenged in this area include:

- Recognizing and appreciating whatever job the animal in your household is doing
- Reassigning jobs when big changes are made in a household to help the animal retain a sense of security
- Letting new animals know that they are loved
- Allowing moments for the animal at the bottom of the pecking order among its species members to just breathe and be themselves

- Finding activities that help the animal gain a strong sense of self and its relationship with you
- Allowing the animal to express itself through play and other joyful activity
- Providing exercise, play, laughing, good food, and clean water to support the animal's health

The Fourth Chakra: The Heart and Unconditional Love

For Humans

The human fourth chakra sits at the chest in the heart center. It's the center of love, universal love, unconditional love, and it reflects when our heart is open or closed. It also reflects forgiveness. This area governs our emotional expression and our ability to nurture others, including animals. It holds our hopes and dreams and the experience and expression of pride.

Physically, this chakra governs our heart, lungs, bronchial tubes, upper back, shoulders, and breasts. The rib cage houses and protects those organs, which are very tender, emotional in nature, and life affirming.

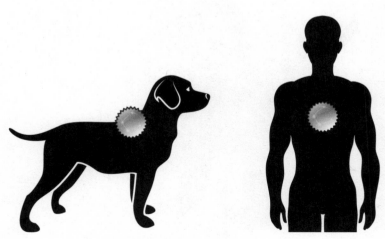

FIGURE 7 Fourth chakra—color, green

Lung and heart disorders are associated with the fourth chakra, as of course is breast cancer. Heart murmurs, asthma, and allergies are all centered here as well.

The fourth chakra can house a broken heart, yet it is a place for all love, not just romantic relationships. As we age, many of us contract in this area to protect our heart or lungs. In Traditional Chinese Medicine, the heart represents joy, while the lungs represent grief. In yoga, when we bend forward and over, we protect these organs, and in doing so, we are protecting the past and our pain. When we do yoga poses that expand the chest, we open our heart to the future.

Self-nurturing is one of the greatest gifts you can give to your fourth chakra. Prayer, meditation, sacred rituals, and taking time to experience joy, along with just plain old breathing, can bring wonderful benefits to your heart center.

For Animals

This is an area of unconditional love for animals too, as well as a nurturing center. As in humans, this area is associated with diseases of

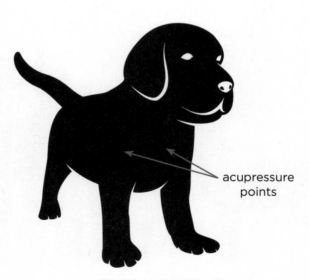

acupressure points

FIGURE 8 The K27 points

the heart and lungs, such as congestive heart failure, lung cancer, and pneumonia (taking the grief on for us). Asthma and allergies live here too as part of the fourth chakra's story.

This area gets sore and breaks down when the animal has a weak hind end; it becomes part of a pattern to compensate for that weakness. The shoulders and necks of dogs that have lost the use of their hind ends can be rock hard, like armor. These are the dogs that carry the world on their shoulders.

Emotional armor can also accumulate in this area in animals that have been handed off to many homes. Some animals actually do die of a broken heart. Animals that have been through many homes frequently could use a good old-fashioned shoulder-and-neck rub.

The K27 points are a great place to massage when there are fourth chakra issues. These acupressure points are located on the chest below the throat at the base of the collar bones and act as the master points for all of the organs. This area alone is a great place to concentrate on when you are introducing a new animal into your home.

In horses, an ill-fitting saddle at the withers (the ridge between the shoulders on four-legged animals) is very common. Continuing the theme of horses having many homes and many jobs, this area is very susceptible to saddle challenges.

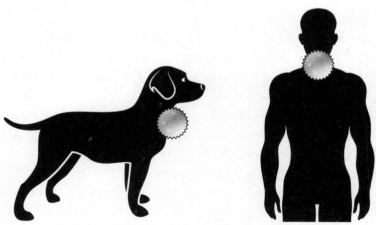

FIGURE 9   Fifth chakra—color, blue

Just as self-nurturing, time, and sacred rituals are good for humans, these are great things to build into our animal companions' day too, particularly if this area is breaking down due to aging. Creating a new ritual or taking the time to enjoy your companion can have huge benefits.

The Fifth Chakra: Creative Expression

For Humans

The fifth chakra is centered in the throat and mouth. It is the area of choice and free will, creative expression, spiritual expression, and our ability to follow our dreams or carry through with our will. Energetically, it can represent speaking the word, or speaking our truth. It is the center of Divine expression.

The fifth chakra is associated with the throat, thyroid and other glands, teeth, gums, parathyroid, trachea, hypothalamus, esophagus, and the vertebrae of the neck. It does not relate to a major organ; instead, it is exposed.

All these glands are part of the endocrine system. In Chinese medicine the endocrine system is associated with the energy of the kidney and the kidney meridian.

For Animals

For our animal friends, this area symbolizes expression and their creativity. Physically, they share the same associations with this chakra that I've just described for humans. Thyroid, teeth, gum, and neck issues all live in this center.

This is the area where we find hypothyroidism in horses and dogs and hyperthyroidism in cats. These conditions affect moods and result in all sorts of skin and hair disorders.

Many animals suffer from jammed necks or severe tightness in this area that goes largely undetected. Tension here can even lead to seizures, and jammed necks pushing into the cranial bones can cause some types of aggression.

When we talk about this being the center for expression, it is certainly the chakra I look at most with regard to aggression. In the course of an initial animal communication session, I try to decipher whether an aggression issue is

- the result of a past trauma (and the animal is therefore reacting in self-defense)
- the result of a physical impingement in the neck or facial bones
- a thyroid issue

Once I know what the issue is, the course to alignment becomes clear to me.

A jammed neck can alter the placement of the facial bones. When that happens, even the alignment of the spine—from head to tail—can change. It's like walking around with an impenetrable shield that limits mobility. This can be accompanied by headaches and other ailments that make the animal feel out of sorts and irritable. In the case of a prey animal, like the horse, it can even affect eyesight.

By definition, thyroid issues mean irritability, and purebreds have a natural predilection for thyroid issues. Sudden weight gain or loss, moodiness, and other temperamental behavior are also strong indications that thyroid levels are off.

WHY DOES YOUR CAT PURR?

Purring is believed to come from vocal folds or cords. While this expression has no anatomical or physical presence in the body, if you hold a purring cat and feel it, the strongest source of the purr is the fifth chakra. Purring can be about food, but it is also very much a loving expression. In fact, studies have shown that purring is actually healing; the low-frequency vibration is said to help build bone density, heal the heart, and is linked to weight loss.

The Sixth Chakra: Intuition

For Humans

The sixth chakra sits on the forehead and is often called the third eye. It is here where we can access all that is seen and unseen. It is the seat of intuition and the site of the thinning of the veil—access to the other world.

The sixth chakra governs the pineal and pituitary glands, the brain, eyes, ears, nose, and nervous system. It is concerned with neurological disorders, learning disabilities, tumors, strokes, and seizures. It also involves the sinus area.

Energetically, when we dream, it is the sixth chakra that leads us through the man- or woman-made movie. Shamanic lore sees the pineal gland as the gateway to the soul or a meeting place between psyche and soma, soul and body.

WORK ON YOURSELF TO HELP YOUR ANIMALS

In the Animal Alchemy weekend workshop I teach, we work on ourselves before we work on the animals. Quite frequently, when I get to the clearing of the third eye, I get such a yummy feeling that it takes me a moment to come back into the

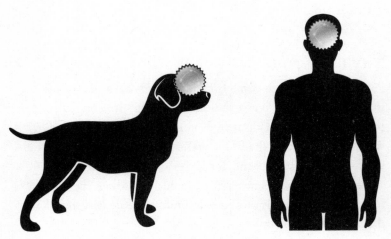

FIGURE 10   Sixth chakra—color, indigo

room! Looking upward toward your third eye with your eyes shut has a hypnotic effect. This is a great place to focus your attention when trying to calm yourself, meditate, or prepare to communicate with animals.

For Animals

The sixth chakra in animals covers the ears, nose, eyes, brain, all of the nervous system, and the pineal gland. A breakdown in this chakra can cause a cat to lose its sense of smell, which can mean the end of its appetite and, worst of all, the end of the cat.

Older dogs get vestibular disease, and that too can mean the end of their life—but sometimes they mysteriously recover. This is a neurological disorder that completely messes with balance and spatial orientation, causing the dogs to feel as if the room is constantly spinning. Again, an issue with the sixth chakra is often involved. This horrible disease can be cured with acupuncture, a change in diet, massage, and herbal remedies. With treatment, a dog that seems like she is at the end of her life can suddenly stand up as if nothing had happened and go on to live happy, healthy years in a very normal way.

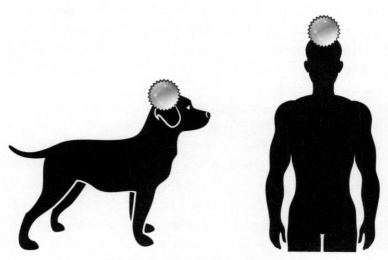

FIGURE 11 Seventh chakra—color, violet

Horses that spook a lot may have had a head injury that moved the cranial bones and the placement of the eye in the socket. In this case, their vision is so different that they don't trust what they see.

In this energy center we find the ability to be seen or unseen—cats have an uncanny ability to become invisible. When you look for a cat and call it, sometimes you can look for it in particular spot, look away, and then look back at that spot to find that the cat is inexplicably there.

The Seventh Chakra: Connection to God/Spirit/Source/Universe

For Humans

The seventh, or crown, chakra sits at top of the head in humans. It governs the entire skeletal and muscular system. It is also the portal to the Divine; it is said that openness here defines the openness one has for the gifts of the Divine. If this chakra is closed, we may feel doubt or forgotten by God.

For Animals

The seventh chakra is at the top of the head in animals too and is also considered the center of connection to the Divine. For some animals, the top of the head may be their most protected spot, and they may feel threatened by a human hand coming toward it. This could be the result of a traumatic event, such as a prior owner swatting a dog over the head with a newspaper.

A lot of animals that have been hit on the top of the head lose faith, so to speak, and are constantly waiting for the other shoe to drop or the next knock on their noggin. For other animals, this is the most delicious place to be scratched.

The top of the head is not just a center of connection to the Divine; it also represents an animal's faith—in us and in other beings. The seventh chakra is also pure, unadulterated faith in existence. Animals don't intellectualize their connection to the Divine; it just is. They are grounded and divinely connected at the same time. In many ways we represent the

Divine to them, so when human hands have hurt this area, an animal's trust in the Divine is shattered. This is an important place to work with to help animals recover their sense of faith in the world.

The beauty of an animal's Divine connection is that they never go to war over it. They don't get possessive about their Divine connection, and they aren't competitive about it. They don't show off how much God has blessed them. They don't create conditions around their Divine connection. In all the time I have been working with animals, no one has ever called me over because of a religious war between two dogs in a household.

This natural divinity is, in part, what draws us to animals. Either we are experiencing fallout from damage to this chakra and we want to make it better for such animals, or we are drawn in by the purity of spirit animals otherwise exhibit, their loyalty and joy regardless of whether it's a sunny day, the paycheck came in, or the rent is due in a few days. We are forever in awe of the knowingness and devotion to Spirit in animals.

What Chakras Teach Us about Our Animals

All of our amazing human achievements, all of our moving human stories, all of our evolution on this planet have involved thought and a myriad of feelings, compounded over time by experience. But a deer or a fox or a rooster can be here *just because*. We really have no place to put that in our calculating brains, our egos, and our thoughts. We have to identify in human terms. We can find no justification or purpose for that deer or fox or rooster. Too often, we conclude that these animals must be here *for us*. But looking at animals energetically, including their chakras, can help us bypass our calculating minds and work with animals as they are—just because.

Humans becoming aware of the chakras can have a profound impact on animal healing. We see that challenges can become energetically embedded in their systems and are not easy to overcome unless these power centers are attended to on a regular basis. When a challenge becomes a pattern and goes unnoticed or is not taken care of by humans, it becomes a "kick me" sign on their backs. The pattern, whether it is behavioral, structural, or physical, becomes their Achilles heel. It is what gets a dog or a cat sent to another home or a horse sent down the road to slaughter.

Really keeping a keen eye on any physical injuries that continually crop up or the emotional or behavioral situations that come forward can clue you in to which chakra is weak and needs support. It will help you travel down the physical, emotional, and spiritual journey to true healing. And any time you facilitate healing for your animals in this way, you are blessed with a little grace yourself.

EXERCISE Using a Pendulum

An interesting exercise you can do with one of your animal friends is to take a pendulum and hold it over the animal's chakras. Take note of whether the pendulum goes in a circular motion or back and forth, and if it's going in a circle, in what direction it is spinning (clockwise or counterclockwise). If you write down what you find, you can note the shift as you apply some of the healing techniques in the next few chapters.

The Energetic Systems of Traditional Chinese Medicine (TCM)

The overall umbrella of Traditional Chinese Medicine (TCM) includes acupressure and acupuncture. Both are tools you can use after a diagnosis has been determined. In TCM, the diagnosis itself is much more complicated than running blood work or taking an x-ray, as is commonly done in Western medicine. Yet it is also much more complete, encompassing many subtle energetic aspects of the individual, including the following:

- The elements: fire, earth, metal, water, wood, each of which is associated with specific organs
- A male (yang) and a female (yin) aspect of opposites

- The meridian system, a map of the body that is also associated with the organs and other features
- Organ profiles that create an understanding of related emotions
- Climate: heat, wind, humidity, dryness, and cold, which help distinguish whether there is too much or not enough of any one of these, giving clues about how to fine-tune the energy

This combination helps inform you as a practitioner about the personality of a patient, making you better able to treat the body, mind, and spirit of an animal when an illness occurs. It also helps keep the animal balanced as a preventative measure. The entire science is holistic and integrative in its approach.

Traditional Chinese Medicine is a big subject—countless volumes have been written about it. In our discussion here about energetic systems, I'll touch on the diagnostic components I just outlined and the differences between acupressure and acupuncture. I'll also offer an overview of why TCM is one of the leading healing methods I use.

TCM works on everything from pain management to boosting the immune system and everything in between, including clarity, focus, recovery from injury, and much more. This system of medicine and healing, part science and part art, is more than five thousand years old. Acupuncture uses needles (thus "puncture") and requires that you be a veterinarian to work on animals. This is a regulated practice, and continuing education is required for the veterinarians who use it. Acupressure, on the other hand, uses pressure, and anyone can practice it on animals. Many books, DVDs, and programs of study can orient you to these techniques.

An Integrated Approach

TCM looks at the well-being of the animal from a variety of viewpoints. This chart summarizes how some of them fit together: elements, emotions, meridians, yin versus yang, and climate.

These elements make up the constitution of the animal, conferring its personality and proclivities. Understanding how the elements show up in health and behavior will not only help you understand why your animal has frequent eye runniness (related to the element wood), for example, but also help you understand why the animal responds as it does to the training process. All of the elements can face threats, and every animal has a weaker, or more challenged, organ system.

Element/Organ	Emotion	Meridian	Yin	Yang	Climate
Fire Heart and Small Intestine	Joy	Pericardium and Triple Heater	Heart/ Pericardium	Small Intestine/ Triple Heater	Heat
Metal Lung and Large Intestine	Grief	Lung/Large Intestine	Lung	Large Intestine	Dry
Wood Liver and Gallbladder	Anger, Liver; Frustration, Gallbladder	Liver and Gallbladder	Liver	Gallbladder	Wind
Earth Spleen, Pancreas, and Stomach	Worry, Spleen; Sympathy, Pancreas; Pensiveness, Stomach	Spleen, Pancreas, and Stomach	Spleen/ Pancreas	Stomach	Humidity
Water Kidney and Urinary Bladder	Fear	Kidney and Urinary Bladder	Kidney	Urinary Bladder	Cold

Elements and Their Constitutions

The "personalities" of the elements and their associated organs and meridians are really more like preferences. Our animals embody these preferences. Of course, there is crossover in that the elements interact in various ways and no animal is any single type. (Also, it should be noted that while horses don't have gallbladders, they still have the energy of the gallbladder meridian.) Now, let's look at the elements in turn.

Fire

Connected to the circulatory system and the heart, this element houses the *Shen,* or Spirit. A dog or a cat with a fire constitution is the happiest thing you've ever seen, bouncing with joy. This is the dog that pees out of excitement, the cat that bounces off the walls like Spiderman—just because—or the horse that is eager to see you and have you around. This level of excitement can tip in the other direction toward nervousness. Animals with this constitution are very sensitive and love to be adored.

In these animals, the small intestine can fire up the enzymes. Overheating the animal or overworking its heart should be avoided. The body part to particularly look at is the tongue.

The season associated with the heart and small intestine is summer, and their active time of day is eleven a.m. to three p.m. The pericardium and triple heater meridians share the summer season and are most active between seven p.m. and eleven p.m.

Metal

Metal is associated with the lung and large intestine meridians. The lung is connected to the Wei Qi, which regulates circulation and prevents climates (wind, damp, cold, etc.) from entering where they don't belong. A dog, cat, or horse with a metal constitution may have had a proclivity for upper respiratory ailments as a baby. This animal might grieve losses a little longer and reflect or absorb the grief of the household. A metal dog or cat would be a soft yet solid presence in the household, loving yet serious. It will also uphold rules and accept human leadership in training while remaining slightly distant. The lung and large intestine meridians are also connected to skin and body hair and open into the nose. The season of metal is autumn, and its active time is from three a.m. to seven a.m.

Wood

Wood is associated with the liver and gallbladder. The liver is in charge of blood flow and tissue. Its emotion is anger. A wood animal could be frustrated, moody, aggressive, and maybe even possessive. Such a dog or cat has its own set of rules and may come off as aloof. A horse would be of the "my-way-or-the-highway" type. This animal may be very athletic. The other body parts associated with the liver and gallbladder are the eyes, tendons, ligaments, and genitals. Animals with runny eyes, hot spots, or itchy skin are wood element animals to some degree. The season of wood is spring, and its power time is from eleven p.m. to three a.m.

Earth

Earth is associated with the spleen, pancreas, and stomach. In TCM, the spleen is more than just a blood and immune center; it is paired with the pancreas because it regulates the blood sugar and breakdown of food in general. An earth animal is your steady, go-to guy. This is the cat that lives to eat and probably doesn't need to hunt. This is the horse you can put a beginner on. This is the dog that is not too ambitious on a walk and waits to sit on the couch to watch *Dancing with the Stars* with you—with a treat, of course. This animal may put on a little weight! It loves everyone and is good with kids. The earth animal can worry or be pensive. The other body part associated with earth is the muscles. The season is late summer, and the time associated with earth is seven a.m. to eleven a.m.

Water

Water is paired with the kidney and bladder. Kidney holds the *jing*, or essence of the animal. As a life force it stores the karma for that body and the inheritance of energy from the ancestors. The kidney is in charge of metabolism. The water dog, cat, or horse lives in perpetual fear; it needs coaxing. A water cat might live under the bed during dinner parties. The water dog barks with the ruff of its neck flared up like an Elizabethan collar. The water horse is rather spooky. Yet these animals are usually very athletic and can be great performers if they have guidance. The kidney rules over bones, marrow, teeth, and genitals. The season is winter, and the time is three p.m. to seven p.m.

Let me emphasize again that there is crossover among these types; no animal stays in one element forever. These energetic systems are constantly in motion as one feeds into the other. When fire burns, it creates soil—earth—and earth moves into metal. Water flows and feeds wood. Sometimes these elements clash or are misdirected, leading to an obstruction of the natural flow of chi, or energy. TCM observes that natural flow and rhythm and facilitates and creates opportunities for the body to right itself by using that natural flow and rhythm.

The Eight Principles of Energy Flow

Eight opposing principles—four sets of two—can assist us in understanding the locations, qualities, or quantities involved in an animal's state:

- Yin and Yang—Yin is the less active, cooling, more feminine energy, as well as the energy of submission. Yang is the heat, the quality of inflammation and fever. It is male and active, if not aggressive.

- Cold and Hot—Cold is like yin energy. This can be a cold chill, coldness moving through the body, or a very calm being. Hot is similar to yang but not as persistent. These animals feel hot, can blow off steam like a volcano, and get swollen glands.

- Exterior and Interior—Exterior: approaching or experiencing an illness at the exterior of the body. Have you ever had the sense that you were off but not submitting to an illness? An example would be if you were slightly run down and dragging but didn't quite catch the flu. The exterior quality is an acute condition with very little fallout. Interior: an illness that is slower and more insidious, more a chronic condition with deep tentacles.

- Excess and Deficiency—Excess means too much: too much water could become edema; too much heat could become inflammation. Deficiency means not enough—as with fatigue or lethargy.

As with the interplay of elements, no animal is always yin or always hot or always in deficiency. Energy is fluid. The environmental influences of wind, dampness, dryness, and summer heat also help determine the nature of a condition and how to treat it.

Vital Essences

There is yet another layer in TCM: the vital essences. These are *jing*, which is our DNA, our heredity, and derived from the kidney; *qi*, also known as chi, which refers to the life force and is contained in bodily fluids (including tears, lymph, urine, and joint fluid); and *shen*, which is Spirit and mind and is both metaphysical and psychological.

∎ ◼ ∎

Elements, principles, meridians, environmental influences, and vital essences—it can all be a bit overwhelming for the layperson. But you can delve into this knowledge as little or as much as you like. Meanwhile, don't think you need to understand it all before you can actually use acupressure to stimulate your cat's nervous system while you're lying on the floor together. Your intuition already knows a lot. And if you want to take advantage of all of the subtleties and complex understandings of TCM, find a TCM practitioner—an acupuncturist DVM.

A TCM Approach to Foods

Like TCM itself, all the ways to feed your dog, cat, or horse based on the elements could fill several books. But setting up a diet according to your animal's needs, based on the organs and elements, is another facet of creating wellness or relaxation. It's best to consult a nutritionist or a holistic vet to create a whole plan, but there are some small things you can do on your own to contribute to your animal's wellness and energy in general.

For example, my dog Olivia, a border collie cross who is now twelve, is a solid citizen. As a puppy, she was as hyperactive as they could be. She raced around on walks with me, went on runs with my then husband, and was always playing with my stepkids. All of that activity was never enough to wear her down! Then one day I was talking to my good friend who is a holistic vet and casually mentioned the raw food I was giving Olivia. When I got to the part about adding oatmeal, I realized even before my friend pointed it out that oats are by nature heat producing. And there I was with a fire dog who was also hormonal (pre-spaying)! It clicked for me that Olivia needed cooling foods.

If you have an earth horse, you might want to add oats. An aging couch potato dog might like the oats too. Although I'm not a huge fan of grains for dogs, there's wisdom in adding a little heat, a little get up and go, when needed.

"You are what you eat" is a great way to approach diet. If we think of how busy a chicken is, its food isn't what we'd want to feed an animal that's already bouncing off the walls, though it might be good for a slower-moving animal. The slow-moving cow, sheep, or bison are better food to fuel the hyperactive dogs and cats.

Including TCM principles with a species-specific diet will bring health benefits to your animals and heart benefits to you because you will feel great knowing you are doing right by your animals! See the Resources section at the end of this book for more great information on nutrition.

The Meridians

We talked briefly about meridians earlier. Starting with a basic understanding of the meridians is a great way to dip your toe into the huge body of knowledge in TCM. You can literally trace the flow of energy. If you were to place your hand on the top of your dog or cat's head and run it across the back to the end of the tail and feel the energy flowing, could you distinguish between sections? Is the energy flow even? Do you feel heat? Do you feel cold spots? Are you aware of where things seem stuck? Like acupuncture, acupressure is designed to move the energy along—it's something you can influence yourself.

Think of a flowing river. It has a life force of its own; it moves forward. When a big boulder falls into the water, this creates a disturbance in the river's pattern, and the water has to go around it. This is what an illness or injury is to the physical system. The meridians have the ability to move the energy back into balance, and you can help in this rebalancing by working with the meridians.

With the exception of the Conception and Governing Vessels, all the meridians are connected to the organs. The meridians are either yin or yang in their influence, and they are all in subtle yet profound communication with the corresponding organ.

Again, with the exception of the Conception and Governing Vessels, all the meridians start or end at either the sides or the fronts of the front and back feet.

- The lung meridian (yin) starts on the inside of the front paw or hoof and comes up to the chest area.

- The large intestine (yang) starts on the front of the paw or hoof and comes up the front legs, through the neck, and up to the nose.

- The spleen meridian (yin) starts on the fourth toe, or dewclaw, or at the second toe on the hind foot and travels up the inside of the hind legs, across the bottom of the torso, up to the area that would be like an armpit, and then toward the withers. It connects on the hind feet with its male counterpart, the stomach.

- The stomach meridian (yang) starts under the eye, comes down to the mouth, travels up to the ear and then back down on the belly, and ends on the inside of the back legs.

- The heart (yin) meets up with the spleen meridian in the armpit and follows down the inside of the front legs.

- The small intestine (yang), on the other side of the foot from the heart meridian, follows up the outside of the front leg, up the shoulder, and up the temporomandibular joint to the ear.

- The pericardium meridian (yin) is on the inside of the front legs, meeting up at the chest where it also meets the kidney meridian. The pericardium is the thin layer that protects the heart. This meridian has an energetic component in that it is the literal and energetic protector of the heart. The pericardium meridian is used to promote joy.

- The triple heater (yang) starts on the front of the front paw or hoof, goes up the front of the leg, up the shoulder, up the neck, over the top of the ear, and down to the outside of the eyes. This meridian is not associated with an organ. Just as it suggests, the triple heater (along with the kidney) is responsible for metabolism and regulating the entire system.

- The liver (yin) meridian meets the gallbladder meridian on the foot, travels up the inside of the hind legs and around the belly (on either side), and ends on the lower rib cage.

- The gallbladder (yang) meridian starts on the hind legs, travels up the outside of the leg and up to the torso and on either side of the lower part of the left hind leg, and follows up the shoulder and neck, making quite a squiggly trail between the eyes and the ears.

- The Conception Vessel (yin) starts right under the tail and moves up the midline on the belly to the top of the bottom lip. It is not associated with an organ.

- The Governing Vessel (yang) starts right under the tail, comes up over the back up to the head, and ends between the nose and the top of the mouth of the animal. It is not associated with an organ, yet it is connected to and with all of the yang organs and meridians.

- The kidney meridian (yin) starts at the main pad of the hind paws, follows up the inside of the hind legs, and trails up the belly and up to the chest. It parallels the Conception Vessel.

- The bladder or urinary meridian (yang) begins at the inside of the eyes on both sides, parallel with the Governing Vessel. It then follows down the back and down the hind quarters and ends on the outside toe. If you only learn about one meridian, the bladder meridian is the fascinating one to study. We will focus on it in Part II, as it contains associated points for all of the organs. These can not only help in healing but also indicate where there is an imbalance in general or an imbalance associated with a particular organ.

As you start learning to work with acupressure points, you will find that they are like a slight depression, a little dip. If you follow a good chart along the bladder meridian, moving from one association point to the next, you might get an idea about what could be challenging your animal. A flinch, a small movement, or even a skin twitch can tell you that something may be going on in the associated organ there.

To be sure that the response you're getting isn't just muscle soreness, using your good chart, you can follow along the abdomen of the animal to the alarm points to see if you find the same sensitivity at the association points. If just the association point is sensitive, that indicates a blockage of energy. If both the association and the alarm points are sensitive, that could indicate something going on with that organ.

■ ◼ ■

But more about working with the points later. Now I'm very excited for you to turn the page and begin Part II, where you'll learn about the many modalities and treatments you can use in energy healing for animals. We'll start with some bodywork options in chapter 6.

Part II

Energy-Healing Modalities

■ ▪ ■

In Part II of this book, you'll get an overview of animal energy-healing modalities, techniques, and technologies. As you review this section, keep in mind that the entire physical being is a series of energy systems that both connect with one another and are heavily influenced by other systems in the body as well as the physical and emotional environments.

Let's take a super pedestrian look at the physical body. Let's think of it as a state: as though your dog or cat or horse—or even you—are a very small version of, say, Colorado or Rhode Island. The skeletal system forms the state's foundation; that's solid rock. The nervous system serves as the central electrical and communication grid for the state. Then we have the circulatory system, the vast network of highways that transport blood everywhere it needs to go—which is pretty much everywhere. The lymphatic system contains the back roads of the state—some paved, some gravel, some dirt—which carry less familiar but no less vital fluids through the system.

The muscular system? Well, that's a blue-collar industry, the nuts and bolts of commerce, while the respiratory system is a white-collar sector, also essential to production but more refined in how it works. A state's population ebbs and flows, of course, and it corresponds to the reproductive system. The skin is the landscape you see on the surface, with all its curves and angles and shadows. What about the energy plant and a waste department? You get a twofer there: the digestive system, which processes fuel and eliminates what's not used. And then there's the endocrine system, which I like to think of as the state capital because it reports to all the other departments. Each organ is a presiding statesman, complete with staff, whose charge is to work with the other organs to make improvements and solve problems. The staff is especially important: for every great organ, there has to be a great backup system. The memos that constantly travel between dignitary and staff? They would be the hormones, making sure everybody has the latest news. These systems all work perfectly together when an animal or a person is in good health—that would be a well-run state full of happy citizens.

So why describe the physical body this way? Because it's easy to relate to. Let's say you're a person with a dog that suffers from arthritis. You don't need a degree in anatomy or physiology in order to think up some of the ways you might give your pet relief. You mostly need a sense of how things flow when the ship of state is sailing well. A basic understanding of how systems work together as a whole, including the influence of emotions and the environment, is a big help as you approach healing modalities.

In this section of the book, it's crucial to look at your animal's body in its entirety—the entire New Jersey or Wisconsin. For instance, you wouldn't single out acupressure as the go-to thing if you want to help a dog with arthritis. Acupressure will help, but you also need to explore whether the digestive, immune, and endocrine systems are contributing to the inflammation, as well as the emotional state of the dog and its household.

Often, when we're talking about health challenges, we're talking about the body and energy body being stressed, and there are hormonal challenges involved in stress. Remember: everyone—including animals—responds to stress differently at different times. If you're seeing anxiety, aggression, fear, depression, or grief in your animal, it's a sure sign it's living with some serious stress and is in high fight-or-flight mode. Now, a wild duck that faces stress—say, the sudden appearance of a bobcat at the edge of the pond—can fly off. Animals in our homes or barns can't do that. They trust us to take care of them. Without the option of just taking off, they can experience stress in ways that are similar to how we respond to chronic stress, setting a mental loop of whatever stresses us on endless replay. The trick is to interrupt that loop.

When we (people and animals) go into stress/fight/flight/fright, the adrenal glands say, "Uh oh! Uh oh! Uh oh!" and they produce adrenaline. The physical body gets extra energy to handle the situation and goes into overdrive. Meanwhile, norepinephrine is released from the adrenal glands and the brain to create high alert.

All this extra energy flying around has to come from somewhere, from other places where it's been doing helpful work, like healing an old wound or bolstering the immune system. So you're sapping the healthy system, and all the while the stress hormone, cortisol, is shooting off like fireworks. And this is how it goes. For some beings, this is actually how it goes all day long.

Bottom line: for any number of reasons, many of the animals in our homes aren't living with the full degree of safety and harmony that could be present for them, and it's stressing them out. We can go a long way toward mitigating some of their illnesses by addressing this. It starts with us.

This second part of the book offers many ideas to help balance your animal's system and your household. They are simply a few ideas, but there are a million out there! Be creative. And remember: none of these can substitute for a qualified veterinarian, trainer, or behaviorist. This is a team effort.

6

Energy Healing
through Bodywork

Our perfect companions never have fewer than four feet.
COLETTE

Touching our animals is a great way to effect healing, but it isn't beneficial only for them. Most of us know how comforting touching or petting an animal can be, and science has shown some of the health and stress-reducing benefits for us, including easing blood pressure. So as we dive into our discussion of bodywork techniques for working with animals, you can be assured that everyone will mutually benefit from your "physician, heal thyself" bodywork experience! Bodywork brings relaxation, increases circulation and oxygen in the blood, helps ease chronic pain, and is a wonderful preventative technique. It also deepens the bond between you and your companion.

Let's begin by laying out some simple overviews of a variety of wonderful modalities. For some, you may want to seek the help of a trained professional as well, while others are simple techniques you can do at home.

Bodywork Overview

Modality	Needs a professional practitioner	Is this a technique with a certification program that I could take?	Requirements	Could I learn it over a weekend for fun?	Could I try it at home with minimal info?
Animal Chiropractic	Yes	No	Must be a veterinarian or a chiropractor	No	No
Bowen Technique	Yes	Yes	Massage therapy credential in order to touch humans in most states	Yes, the basics	No
Water Therapy	Yes	Yes	Canine massage or acupressure	No	No
Acupuncture	Yes	Must be a veterinarian	Must be a veterinarian or a chiropractor	No	No
Animal Massage	Yes	Yes	Lots of hours in the program and tests	Yes, the basics	Very, very basic
Myofascial Release	Yes	Yes, usually included in massage schools	No	Yes	Yes

Animal Chiropractic

What is it? Chiropractors carefully manipulate joints to restore correct alignment, which is believed to improve nerve function throughout the body. Through examination, practitioners aim to identify and then treat subluxations, or misalignments of joints.

Like humans, animals defend themselves from pain, creating compensation patterns. The older they get the more entrenched these physical patterns can become. Injuries from prior years can also create unnatural postures or gaits. Sometimes the root cause of a behavior change is being out of alignment, but our animal companions can't tell us that they are in pain or compromised in some way.

Who does this help? Super active, athletic, injured, and aging animals. Chiropractic adjustments are wonderful preventative care, particularly as our animals age. And chiropractic adjustments are necessary for active and athletic horses. Just imagine the physical dynamic at work when a horse's spine moves one way and the spine of the rider on top of it moves another way. Add to this that the rider might be guiding this large animal at a fast pace, jumping over things, doing quick turns on a polo field or in a barrel race, or demanding the precision of dressage—and all the while the horse's spine is bearing the rider's weight and responding to specific muscular demands.

Dogs that do the sport of agility, herding, or any activity that repetitively uses specific muscle groups are good candidates for chiropractic. Dogs that frequently go on long hikes could probably use an adjustment. And let's face it: if you live with a small pack of rowdy dogs, somebody has usually been trampled and could use a little relief.

Cats that think they're superheroes can use some help from chiropractic. You know the one I'm talking about: the cat that jumps off the top of the fridge, tries to climb up the side of the house, or dangles from your drapes. Cats with a history of bladder infections usually need an adjustment as well. Adventurous, devil-may-care cats, who are all about running, chasing, and leaping, can come out of alignment. Sometimes our pets can simply jump off the couch and land wrong, jamming up one of their joints. Chiropractic is a great remedy for that.

Who is qualified to perform this on my animal or to teach me how to do it? Chiropractors (DC) who have trained and certified through the American Veterinary Chiropractic Association (AVCA) or veterinarians (DVM) who have trained and certified through the AVCA. You can also rely upon veterinarians trained and certified in Veterinary Orthopedic Manipulation (VOM). VOM is a healing technology that locates areas of the animal's nervous system that have fallen out of communication. It reestablishes neuronal communication and thus induces healing. Some bodywork and energy balancing work, while not considered chiropractic, have an adjustment component, so there are lots of people who perform this and can teach you simple moves.

Is there anything I can do at home that a chiropractor might do? Generally speaking, there are two things you can do: palpate and stretch. However, unless you're under the wing of someone who has given you homework to practice, it's best to see a professional to get your animal companion in alignment. You don't want to make it worse or injure your pet in a different way.

If you work gently, here are a few techniques you can do and trouble spots to look out for:

Palpating

If you notice a different gait in your dog, cat, or horse, you can gently press along the spine to see if you get a reaction or a muscle spasm. If that happens, you know the animal needs an adjustment. Or let your hands glide along the bladder meridian and notice if there are changes in temperature along the spine or legs. Palpating is helpful even if the problem you see is a difference in your animal's behavior. The animal could be masking pain.

Stretching

If you aren't dealing with a major injury, you can always lift the rib cage gently in a stretch. You can gently move the tail up and down and turn it like a little crank in either direction. You can bring the legs straight out in a stretch. You can move your hands from below the throat down to the chest, as if to ask for a little space between each vertebra in the neck. And you can turn the head to the left and then to the right while holding the body still.

You can always move or turn a horse or a dog to rotate its hind end around the forehand (the front legs) to open up the hips in both directions. Do the same on the hind legs to get the horse or dog to open up the shoulder, pivoting the front end around the relatively still hind end. You can always try any of these stretches with a cat, but you might want to don your combat gear first.

Bowen Technique

What is it? Developed in the 1950s by the late Tom Bowen of Geelong, Victoria, Australia, the Bowen Technique can be quite useful. After serving in World War II, Bowen became interested in ways to alleviate human suffering and began to notice that certain moves on the body had particular effects. Thankfully, someone realized the technique also works beautifully on animals.

A series of hands-on, gentle, rolling moves along the spine and at receptor points for muscles, tendons, and ligaments removes toxins, allowing better muscle tone and an improved range of motion as well as gait. This is one of those therapies that seem to reset the whole system though you seem to be treating one ailment, so there is an overall wellness benefit to this healing work.

Who does it help? Bowen Therapy is great for performance animals and is a wonderful maintenance program for any animal. It's also very beneficial for musculoskeletal conditions, arthritis, post surgery, speeding up recovery from an injury, decreasing inflammation, and relieving stress from thunderstorms. Lymphatic drain and improved circulation are automatic bonuses! Bowen Therapy resets the autonomic nervous system and relaxes the animal into its parasympathetic nervous system. Because it is a "nonforce" technique, this is great for animals that are highly sensitive, have had severe trauma, or are terrified of touch. Bowen can also be helpful for emotional conditions like fear and aggression.

Who is qualified to perform this work or to teach me? There is a vast Bowen network, and the Bowen Practitioner Directory is listed in the back of the book.

Water Therapy

What is it? Like humans, animals benefit from a simple exercise known as swimming. Water therapy mobilizes joints without adding pressure to the joints because it's a non-weight-bearing exercise. It's good for everything from joints to connective tissue (fascia), to circulation, to increasing oxygen. Plus it's fun for both animals and humans! You can make this a playful activity. For example, while your dog chases a ball, he's actually doing a water therapy exercise by simply swimming. Then a therapist can slip in some serious acupressure or massage moves that a ball-obsessed dog wouldn't ordinarily sit through.

Water therapy for horses is usually offered only at very expensive spas or rehab centers, where frequently there is also a treadmill the horses walk and then run on in a long skinny pool. I haven't heard of any cat water facilities yet (see the previous section about combat gear), although certain states are starting to develop dog water therapy programs. Check with your state's holistic doctors for any suggestions.

Who does it help? Water therapy is great for helping the injured athlete return to performance level and for the aging animal that is losing strength or muscle tone. Obviously, dogs with a fear of water aren't going to benefit from this modality; in fact, water may create more stress for them.

Who is qualified to perform this care or to teach me? You can find qualified people at water facilities for dogs and horses.

Is there anything I can do at home? If you have a hot tub or a pool or live near a lake or on the beach, you can get your dog or horse into the water and let them swim. And as long as you aren't compromising your own safety, you can gently try some of the bodywork techniques mentioned in this book. As always, it is best to have a professional get you started.

Acupuncture

What is it? Acupuncture is the main component of TCM (Traditional Chinese Medicine). As I discussed in Part I, TCM is a very complex and complete system that can be used to diagnose and heal the core of an issue. Acupuncture applies very small needles to points along the meridians of the body—a system, as we reviewed, that is not unlike highways dedicated to organs throughout the body, with the acupuncture points being tiny destinations. It is a very holistic and integrative approach. TCM doesn't differentiate between what goes on in the liver of the body and what goes on in the anger of the being.

These acupuncture points may either need to be stimulated or toned down, depending on the condition. A trained acupuncturist truly masters the science and art of this form of healing. If he or she is knowledgeable in Chinese herbs, these may also be prescribed. Chinese herbs are very different from Western ones and can make a world of difference, especially while healing from a major health issue, including vestibular disease in dogs.

Who does this help? Since TCM approaches the whole being, the healing can address a vast array of ailments, from endocrine disorders to digestive problems. It's useful in regulating cardiovascular health and healing an injury. A better question is, what doesn't it help?

Who is qualified to perform this or to teach me? Acupuncture is not for the uninitiated. It must be performed by a veterinarian who has trained and been accredited by the International Veterinary Acupuncture Society. Some chiropractors have a diploma in acupuncture as well. Be wary of anyone who isn't a DVM and claims to be able to do animal acupuncture.

Is there anything I can do at home? Again, if there is a suspected injury, palpating along the spine is an excellent approach. Studying acupressure is the next best thing.

Animal Massage

What is it? Massage helps improve circulation, increase range of motion, deepen relaxation, relieve muscle stiffness and spasms, break up scar tissue from old injuries, and break up the muscle memory in our animal companions. It also promotes emotional healing.

Who does it help? Most of us love a massage. Many of us go for therapeutic reasons, including relaxation, maintenance, and to recover from injuries. Those are all great reasons to find a massage therapist for your animal companion.

It's a fact that any horse that is being ridden could use a massage. If there is any level of competition or repetitive motion—in any discipline—the horse can benefit from massage.

Some of the more tightly wound dog breeds, such as Jack Russells, herding dogs, and the breeds that take their work very seriously, benefit from massage. Of course, the little pocket breeds deserve it just because they're amazing friends and family members. Believe it or not, cats enjoy massage as well. It just won't be as long a session once they catch on to what you're doing to them (even if it's for their own good)!

Who is qualified to perform this or to teach me? Canine, equine, and feline massage therapists are certified through programs much like those a human massage therapist completes. They take hours of anatomy and physiology classes and log in a lot of structured practice. And yes, they can show you certain moves. If you're interested in studying animal massage, I list a massage school in the Resources section at the end of this book. Some states require that equine/canine/feline massage therapists either be licensed veterinary technicians or have completed a human massage course.

Is there anything I can do at home? Your animal will certainly benefit from your intuitive efforts at massage. It might also be worth it to find a canine or equine massage therapist in your area. Most of us in the animal healing field do basic moves while we're watching TV or

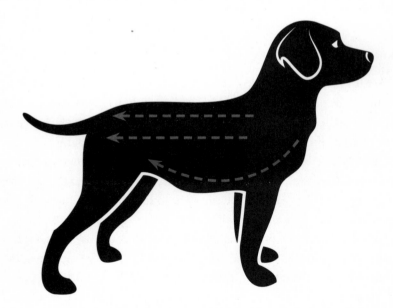

FIGURE 12   A mini ribcage massage, moving from front to flank

reading alongside our animal companion. Your equine friend works so hard for you and will appreciate your massaging sore spots; you should find the time to give back.

EXERCISE   Mini Rib-Cage Massage

Start with your flat hand adjacent and just next to the spine and along the rib cage, and stroke your dog or cat along the rib cage from the shoulder to the flank. Then lower your hand about a half inch and start again at the shoulder and move slowly back the flank. Move your hand under the ribcage at the chest and slowly bring your hand back to the tummy.

If the animal is standing, you can do both sides at the same time, one with each hand. As you come around to stroke the chest through the belly under the rib cage, you can get a good stretch out of the spine. Do this move slowly one more time—really stretching the spine out is excellent.

If the animal can't stand or you are lying down, lift the front leg gently. You can still create the spinal stretch with the slightest amount of pressure.

This is a great little technique for stimulating the organs (especially organs of digestion) and for assessing your companion's body. Your flat hand will detect any lumps or growths. The final stroke from the chest to the stomach also stimulates the heart.

Myofascial Release

What is it? Fascia is the connective soft tissue that covers much of the body like a sheet while also connecting parts of the body. It is part of and protects the muscles, bones, tendons, ligaments, organs, nervous system, and more. So if the energy is off or if there has been an injury, think of that as a ruffling or a wrinkling in this sheet that restricts movement, covering scar tissue. Myofascial release smoothes out the wrinkles.

The practitioner uses some degree of force, not a lot of weight, and may need to use a flat hand, knuckle, or an elbow. The force creates resistance in the injury itself and remains as pressure until the tissue releases. Fascial release allows greater freedom of motion, improving gait and flexibility. It can also remove physical and emotional trauma from specific areas of the body. Scar tissue can be localized and manipulated. When the release is being performed, there is almost a sense that the old injury is "unwinding." This unwinding may bring up the emotion of the injury, and the emotion will be released as well.

Who does it help? Myofascial release is especially beneficial for animals with injuries and scar tissue. It also helps animals that perform repetitive motion, such as horses that jump, perform dressage, or barrel race. It helps dogs who herd or pull carts and aids in their basic agility. It will also help aging dogs that have trouble going to the bathroom. Myofascial release helps cats that like to perch up high and have a long drop down, as well as cats that strain in the litter box.

Who is qualified to perform this or to teach me? Most physical therapists, occupational therapists, massage therapists, cranial sacral therapists, DOs, DCs, and acupuncturists have learned and employ this technique.

Is there anything I can do at home? The best thing you can do yourself is a very light myofascial release. To get the sensation, you might try it with one hand on a scar of your own—or talk a friend into being your guinea pig! I would suggest trying it on a person first (or yourself) because there is an emotional component to the release, and you can get feedback about that.

You could also do the following lightly with a flat hand on an animal companion, but unless you have training, I wouldn't suggest you jump into an old injury on your donkey friend with your elbow.

Here are the steps:

- Put your flat hand on the old injury or scar tissue, and push and elongate the tissue in one direction, using minimal pressure. See if you can sense a pulse. Also see if you get a sense of an emotion associated with the scar tissue. See if you can feel it unwinding as you elongate the tissues. If you don't have a sense one way or another, keep your hand there until you feel complete.

- Now move the old injury or scar tissue back in the opposite direction, creating a little resistance or pressure. Again, see what sensations come up.

- Next, move the injury or scar tissue in a third direction, creating a little resistance or pressure. Again, see what sensations come up. Sometimes this third move can result in the most dramatic pulsing or unwinding. Just be with that for the moment, and then take your hand away.

- Shake both of your hands out as if to rid them of the injury.

Trying this first on an old injury of your own is a great way to get familiar with this technique because you can assess the various sensations for yourself and see what your animal companion might experience. You can feel where the pulsing or energy is the strongest. And then, as the pulsing slows down, you can feel how the sting of the old injury—emotional and physical—has been released. And don't worry that you'll do damage using this gentle technique. You can't hurt scar tissue, and you may even release trapped muscle memory.

∎ ▪ ∎

The next category of modalities I'll introduce you to is what I think of as hands-on energy work. I'll introduce you to these in chapter 7.

7

More Hands-On
Energy-Healing Techniques

Animals are reliable, many full of love, true in their affections,
predictable in their actions, grateful and loyal.
Difficult standards for people to live up to.

ALFRED A. MONTAPERT

The bodywork techniques in the last chapter were mainly structural approaches to energy healing, and while you could do some of the work yourself, most require the skill and knowledge of a professional. The modalities in this chapter are mainly structural too, but they are a little more human-companion friendly. They are also techniques that address emotional as well as physical health. The key to energy healing using these methods is intention.

Acupressure

What is it? I mentioned acupressure in the last chapter on bodywork. Here I'll go into a little more detail because it's a great way to address emotional issues energetically as well. Acupressure and acupuncture are both leading healing methods for managing pain, recovering from injury, boosting the immune system, aiding clarity and focus, and so

Hands-On Energy-Work Overview

Modality	Needs a professional practitioner	Is this a technique with a certification program that I could do?	Requirements	Could I learn it over a weekend for fun?	Could I try at home with minimal info?
Acupressure	Yes and you can learn to do it too with formal training	Yes	None	Yes	Yes
Cranio-Sacral	Yes and you can learn to do it too with formal training	Yes	Massage therapy for humans	Yes	Yes, basic moves
TTouch	Yes	Yes	None	Yes	Yes
Healing Touch for Animals	Yes	Yes	Lots of hours in the program and tests	Yes	Very, very basic

much more. Like acupuncture, acupressure uses pressure points located along the meridians, the energy pathways of Traditional Chinese Medicine that correspond to organs, energy systems, and emotions. As such, it is both a science and an art that dates back more than five thousand years and has proven effective time and time again. Acupuncture uses needles (thus "puncture" in the term—and the reason a lot of training is required), and acupressure uses pressure.

Who does this help? The simple answer is . . . anyone with a body!

Who is qualified to perform this or to teach me? Someone who has studied acupressure from a reputable program (see the Resources section.)

Is there anything I can do at home? Yes. There are books, training courses, DVDs, and more available for those who want to learn this technique. I have listed several of these in the resources section. For now, I'll offer some brief instruction along with a few important points.

Locating the Acupressure Points

It is helpful to have a chart of the main acupressure points when you begin (see the books on acupressure in the Resources section). Then you will know you've located an acupressure point when you feel a slight groove or dip in the area indicated. Your finger will go in a little farther than if you were poking along somewhere else. Once you've found the point, press very lightly; when you are treating an animal, you want to use no more than five ounces of pressure.

Now simply sit and breathe for a moment and feel a sense of connection with that point. If you concentrate on your breath and allow your breath to connect with the breathing pattern of your animal companion, this will give you an even deeper connection with that animal.

If the point is stagnant, you might not feel anything going on there at first. Eventually, the slight sense of a heartbeat should arise. If it doesn't, feeling a pulse at that spot is still the goal—the heartbeat should slowly rise to your fingertips, even if it's faint.

Let me repeat that the pressure you use should be light. With most bodywork (very intense systems like Rolfing being the exceptions), less is more. Animals are already energetic and sensitive, so you don't want or need to come on strong. You don't have to wiggle your fingers around, or really do anything other than just hang out there making contact. Simply allow the energy flowing through that point and whatever you are feeling there to be. Then gently release the pressure. You'll find that the energy meets your touch and then fades.

Things You Can Do at Home

THE BLADDER MERIDIAN

You could spend a lifetime working just with your animal's Bladder Meridian, which runs on either side of and parallel to the spine, from head to tail. That's because even though each of the main organs has a dedicated meridian of its own, the Bladder Meridian contains "association points" that correspond to all of them as well. This meridian is very alive and vital in animals, and working with it alone can ignite a sluggish nervous system. Sometimes, nerves just need a reminder.

The easiest and most effective way to work with the Bladder Meridian is "the bladder sweep." It evens out the animal's energy, and with practice, your hands will get a feel for any heat, coolness, or energy disturbances. A bladder sweep is just as it sounds: you slowly sweep your hand along the meridian, from the forehead all the way to the base of the spine and then down each leg. On the first sweep, take your hand from the top of the head across the back and follow the left hind leg on down to the foot. On the second sweep, start at the forehead and sweep along the meridian down the right leg to the foot. The third sweep starts at the forehead too, but this time, simply follow along the bladder meridian out the end of the tail. (If the animal has a missing limb or a docked tail, sweep down to the end of where the limb or tail would be.)

JING POINTS

There are a variety of points on the meridians: sedation points, tonifying points, association points, and more. Jing points are found at the beginning or the end of a meridian. In dogs and cats, they are found on the sides and tops of the toes, where the nail bed meets the fur, as well as on the bottom of the foot where the pad meets the fur. On the horse, the jing points are right along the coronet band, where the top of the hoof meets the hairline, and there are four of them: front and back, medial and lateral. (On people, they are where the fingernail meets the skin.)

According to TCM, these points stimulate the immune system, and I often work with them on myself. When I get on an airplane, for example, and it looks like I'm fidgeting, I'm actually activating my jing points just in case I'm sitting next to someone with a cold.

To explore jing points on yourself, take a moment and place your right thumb on your left thumb where the nail bed meets the skin. Place about five ounces of pressure there and breathe for five to ten breaths. Next, place your right thumb toward the outside of the left thumb at the nail bed for a few breaths and then toward the inside for a few breaths. What sensations do you feel? When I do this, I immediately have a sense of well-being, and I breathe more deeply. There's a good reason for that: the outside of the thumb is Lung 11 in Traditional Chinese Medicine.

The jing points are also known to aid in circulation. While human jing points are located on our hands and the top of our toes, animals actually stand on some of their jing points. That's why the bottoms of the feet are great places to massage and perform acupressure on dogs and cats, to energize the circulation there. On horses, that area right above the hoof is a great place to massage or to do acupressure because it also ensures circulation to the hoof.

Cranial Sacral Therapy

What is it? Cranial Sacral Therapy (CST) is a subtle, relaxing, noninvasive holistic therapy for your animal companion that helps facilitate its body's natural ability to heal itself. Using their hands, practitioners of CST gently realign the bones in the skull and at the base of the spine to release tension and harmonize the central nervous system.

Your animal's cranial sacral system is made up of the cranium (the bones of the skull), the membranes and fluid surrounding the brain and spinal cord, and the sacrum (at the base of spine). The goal of CST is to help the fluid follow a very natural and succinct rhythm as it flows from the cranium to the sacrum and back again.

Who does it help? CST is particularly helpful in recovering from an accident, correcting posture, or coming back from an illness or major stress that has upset the rhythm of the fluid. The system just needs to be reminded—jump-started back to its natural flow—with hand placement and intention.

Who is qualified to perform this or to teach me? An experienced practitioner can teach you the basic moves, but generally a certified cranial sacral practitioner is your best bet.

Is there anything I can do at home? Yes! Here is a little realignment technique:

1. Sit beside your animal and place your left hand on top of its head and your right hand on top of its sacrum.

2. Imagine that you are balancing out the system between your hands to create a rhythmic flow.

3. See if you have a sense of that fluid that bathes the brain and spine flowing between your hands. When it is up in the head, the bones there expand. Even if you don't feel that happening in your animal's head right now, imagine and act as if you do feel it. Feel your hand respond, lifting slightly, as the bones of the cranium expand. This will take just a few seconds. Then . . .

4. As fluid drains out of the cranium and the cranium contracts, your hand will lower slightly. The fluid will flow toward the sacrum. At this point your hand over the sacrum should experience the slight lifting.

5. Now simply sit with that ebb and flow: the right hand lifting slightly, the left hand lowering slightly, and then the reverse—the left hand lifting and the right hand lowering. Feel the rhythm shift as the fluid moves from head to tail and back again.

One of the keys to doing this very subtle work is *not* to get into your head to try to analyze what's happening. If you don't feel anything at first, pretending works just fine. Create a pretend rhythm. Just being with this energy can remind body, energy, and fluid where it needs to go, so your animal can regain a sense of rhythm.

Just as with TCM, when we think of a disturbance, an injury, or a health challenge our animal is experiencing, we can imagine it as a boulder in a stream, creating a disturbance that causes the water flow to adjust. Our hands are reminding the system how the flow originally went, and the cranial and sacral bones will make subtle shifts under our hands to increase that flow.

Healing Touch for Animals

What is it? Healing Touch for Animals (HTA) was created in the early 1990s by Carol Komitor, a licensed veterinary technician and certified Healing Touch practitioner. The system bridges holistic touch and veterinary medicine in a cooperative model.

HTA is a wonderful blend of the values of touch and intention, and its results can be measured scientifically. The intention of the practitioner is to clear and facilitate physical, emotional, spiritual, and mental health. HTA clears the energy field and energizes the animal at the same time.

In the human world, Healing Touch is now recognized as effective by the medical community and is being employed by many hospitals as part of recovery and maintenance for human patients.

Who does it help? HTA can help any animal feel greater energy. It can promote healing after surgery and affect overall healing of injuries. After a traumatic accident, it helps the animal feel like it's back in its body. HTA also benefits animals experiencing emotional trauma, including being moved to a different home and losing a family member, whether a person or an animal. It helps animals that are going through a career change, such as not fitting into a service dog program, stepping down from being a champion in the show world to simply being a house pet, or going "out to pasture" for a horse. There's almost no end to the energetic benefits of this technique.

HTA brings about a sense of groundedness and well-being, so it's perfect for hyper animals, like those that pitch a fit when getting into a car, making the experience almost intolerable for the human involved. HTA helps the nervous cat going to the veterinarian or the horse that's doing something new, such as its first trail ride. HTA is an excellent aid in training, as it helps insecure and nervous animals.

Who is qualified to perform this or to teach me? There are HTA workshops all over the United States and abroad. An HTA practitioner can show you basic grounding techniques and will bring great benefits to your animal companion with a professional session. To learn the full spectrum of what HTA has to offer, you can turn to some of the resources at the back of this book.

Is there anything I can try at home? Yes! While there are many HTA techniques, the best one to try to give you a sense of the power and simplicity of this technique is vibrational grooming, a way of clearing the energy field. This is a great way to incorporate a little energy work into your daily life, to get grounded yourself and really connect with your animal companion. It's also a wonderful way to get a sense of the animal's energy field and clear away any disturbances.

To do vibrational grooming, simply use your regular grooming tools as an extension of your hand to brush through the animal's energy field. As you groom from the top of the head to the end of the tail, use the grooming tool as an aid to go through more than just hair. Imagine that any debris or congestion the animal may be carrying with them is being brushed away. That simple intention does the work!

TTouch

What is it? TTouch, created by Linda Tellington-Jones, is a type of body-work that's so subtle you can easily find yourself questioning at times whether it's working. Yet it's one of the most powerful and effective techniques ever. It includes many different movements or ways of touching, the most famous being the TTouch little circles. These circular motions awaken the cells; it's as though you're electrifying the cells with your fingers.

Pain, illness, and phobias are stress patterns in the energy system. TTouch shifts these stress patterns and stabilizes the animal in the parasympathetic nervous system mode, which is relaxation. Basically, TTouch "wakes up" the pattern and asks it to be something different, using no more pressure than it takes to simply move the skin around. This form of touch talks to the cellular memory involved in the pattern of illness or pain, in effect saying, "Okay—enough already. Let's repattern this!" If you learn only one technique to turn to at the drop of a hat, this is the magic potion.

Who does it help? I'm not overstating it when I say that TTouch addresses every kind of energetic problem! It helps fearful animals by shifting them from being in fight-or-flight mode to being grounded. It also helps bring an animal in distress back into its body. TTouch works wonders with teething puppies, and it's excellent both post surgery and for recovering from an injury. Arthritis, nerve pain, and hip dysplasia are only a few of the ailments that greatly benefit from TTouch.

TTouch also addresses emotional challenges, such as insecurities from a previous difficult experience (like switching homes), trying something new in training, overexcitement, grief, and achieving some relaxation before a big show or a performance, to name a few specifics.

Who is qualified to perform this and to teach me? There are plenty of places online where you can learn the techniques, as well as books and DVDs. Tellington-Jones also has a wide-ranging group of certified teachers all over the world.

Is there anything I can do at home? Yes! You can do TTouch little circles.

TTouch little circles are small, clockwise circles that are basically one full circle plus a quarter circle. By moving around the body from one circle to the next, you subtly engage the animal's entire energetic system. *Now* the system is listening.

To do the most basic circle, place your resting hand on the animal with a calming intention. Use your index and second finger to create the circles. Like all the other techniques I'm inviting you to try at home, you want to do this with minimal pressure.

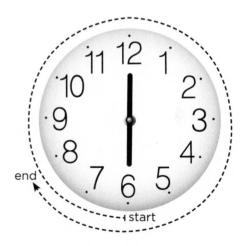

FIGURE 13 With TTouch, you start at 6 o'clock, then go all the way around and past 6 o'clock to 8 o'clock—almost a circle and a quarter

Imagine that the circle is the face of the clock. Start at six o'clock, make a full circle to six o'clock again, and then go past it to eight o'clock—so the movement is a full circle and a teeny bit further. Then release and move on to do another circle, and another, and another, and so on and so on.

The series of circles you do should not create a pattern. Use your intuition, and move randomly. Our purpose here is to repattern the condition, whether physical or behavioral, we want to energetically shift for the animal. The goal is not to create a new pattern but to reset the system.

■ ■ ■

All the techniques I covered in this chapter are very accessible—and very enjoyable for both you and your animal! And as with every method in this book that you can do yourself, the more your practice, the easier it will be to shift your animal's energy. It will be second nature before you know it.

8

Shifting Energy with
Nutrition and Homeopathy

I care not much for a man's religion
whose dog and cat are not the better for it.
ABRAHAM LINCOLN

Nutrition

You might not think of food as a subtle energy technology, but I believe that food is one of the foremost energetic technologies to consider for optimum health and behavior. You can pour vitamin C into your dog, lay him on a crystal bed, and give him a cranial sacral session, but if the food you're feeding him isn't supporting him, you'll probably just break even at best. You won't see the kind of sweeping positive shift you could if you include nutrition in your overall recipe for healing.

What is it? Nutrition is the process of absorbing nutrients in order to grow and maintain health. When the body is truly fed for optimum energy with good nutrition, minerals, and vitamins, any other substances you give your animal, such as herbs or homeopathic remedies, will work that much quicker. Chiropractic adjustments and massage treatments will serve the body longer. The old saying "You are what you eat" is as true for our animal companions as it is for us.

Nutrition, of course, is a vast subject. Countless volumes have been written about it, and I could probably write a full book on the subject myself based on my experience with animals. But I'm not going to outline diets here, nor am I going to review the best pet foods. I list several wonderful books that cover these items in the Resources section of this book. What I will do here is break down some simple things to consider about your animal companion's diet.

My favorite book on this subject is Kymythy Schultze's *Natural Nutrition for Dogs and Cats: The Ultimate Diet.* In it she includes species-specific diets. She uses a pyramid model with the largest section being at the bottom, tapering off to the least needed foods at the top. From the bottom up, it reads: Meat, Bones, Vegetables, and Other (vitamins, minerals, and herbs).

Dr. Pitcairn is on the cutting-edge of revising diets for dogs and cats. He is researching diets with less meat, as it carries contaminates and is not compassionate to the planet.

If you don't feel you can prepare raw food for your animal friend, could you feed prepared raw food? Could you look into the second-best option, cooking for your animal? There are plenty of recipe books available. Last but not least on my list is food out of a bag or can. (Again, see Resources for a website listing of these best foods.)

Here are some things to consider when purchasing prepared food:

- Do you know what's in that bag?
- Do you trust all of the ingredients?
- Do you know where the ingredients came from?
- Was only dog or cat food made in that mill that day? (Or could there have been other things that aren't so great for your animal going through that mill?)
- Are there GMOs (genetically modified organisms) in the ingredients?
- Are there hormones in the meat?
- Was the meat factory farmed?
- Do you know the quality of the soil that the food was grown in?
- Do *you* eat the same thing every day?

If you ask yourself these questions, you can see that trusting the ingredients in bagged or canned food and how it was put together is a really tall order. And the truth is that we are seeing frightening recalls every day.

We also have some very bad practices that lead to our animals' health challenges. We leave food out for cats, for example, more for our convenience than theirs. But isn't kidney disease later on more of an inconvenience? Obviously, dry food doesn't exist in the wild, and cats have to drink a lot of water to counter it. Their kidneys weren't set up for that. Once we realize this, we can put food down for them when they need it, as if they had just ordered it from "our restaurant."

Constant access to dry food also continues to create obesity challenges for our dogs and cats. In the wild they would be hunting: crouching down, running, experiencing a rush of excitement and adrenaline, all the physicality that goes into hunting. By the time a dog or a cat tears into the animal it killed, its digestive enzymes would be prepared for a meal. Now *that* is energy in motion! This is why it's a good idea to consider exercising your animal before you feed it—to engage the enzymes.

The stomach is in constant motion, balancing its pH (potential of hydrogen), which is a dance between acidity and alkalinity. Disease can't live in an alkaline state, so foods and activities that create balanced pH are necessary for good health. Also, the stomach is considered the "second brain." Animals, as we've discussed, are in touch with their instincts, and one of the main vehicles for their instinctual messages is the stomach. A perfect example is the animal that knows well in advance a storm is coming: it feels the barometric pressure change in its stomach.

Then there are the intestines, which are lined with lots of nerve endings that communicate with the autonomic nervous system (the aspect of the nervous system that is in charge of automatic functions, like breathing and blinking). If we feed our animals the wrong foods, they dull the nerve endings and inhibit the animals' natural instincts. The wrong foods also constrain the production of serotonin, which regulates mood; this can contribute to metabolic disorders—and here behavior and health become intertwined. Imagine the stomach, the intestinal tract, and digestion in general serving as a parallel central nervous system with its own operating system. How can we best serve this operating system?

Something else to consider are the levels of minerals in our animal foods. Modern farming practices have depleted the mineral content in the soils where we grow our food, and the resulting foods lack the earth energy of the foods we produced generations ago. This is why finding a way to balance the mineral content in your animal's food—which is the grounding agent for their entire system—is very important. Supplementing with minerals and vitamins is essential. You can think of minerals as roots that ground the body, enabling vitamins to then light up and activate it.

When horses graze in the field, they are eating live food. Yet many horses in our modern world are in barns for much longer stretches than they spend out grazing in a pasture. Horses generally sleep for only four hours in the twenty-four-hour cycle—and even then not all at once—so the motility of their system is set up to eat approximately twenty hours a day. Leaving their stomachs empty for most of the day and feeding them at specific times challenges an operating system built for grazing (and at no time did the prehistoric horse order up food delivered in a bag).

If there is one most important piece of advice I have for you about feeding your animals, it is to feed a species-specific diet. I am personally a fan of raw food for dogs and cats. That said, I also know that some people simply aren't up for preparing raw foods. Fortunately, some new and innovative products have recently appeared on the market: companies that will prepare and send a week's supply, so you don't have to crowd your freezer space, and the food is super fresh. Gone are the days when you had to go on a scavenger hunt yourself to find all the raw ingredients to feed your dog or cat—and even when you found them, combining meat and bone meal and the right amount of vegetables made a giant mess. Talk about daunting!

It's important to invest some time and energy into feeding your animal friends, though not only for their sake but also for yours. Good nutrition will save you in veterinary bills as well as heartache, while instilling peace of mind. Knowing that you are feeding your animals the very best is great energetic medicine for you! We need to see food as fuel: what kind of fuel are we giving our beloved animals—the cheap, the middle of the road, or the premium? Is what we're feeding going to help their system or weigh them down?

Traditional Chinese Medicine understands food as fuel and takes the expression "you are what you eat" quite literally. What is the energy of the food itself contributing to a health situation you deal with on a daily basis? TCM practitioners look at allergies, for example, and see a lot of activity such as aggravation, itching, and scratching. According to TCM theory, feeding chicken—an animal that busily scratches at the ground all day—to your itchy friend could aggravate the situation. Think about it: a chicken never stands still. The same principle applies to the high-energy young dog or a dog that was bred to work but doesn't live on a farm. In both cases it would be better to feed lamb, beef, or bison as main meals. On the other hand, if you have a lethargic dog or an elderly dog, chicken is a great choice.

Who does it help? Everyone. For healthy animals, good nutrition is a preventative measure. For animals that come into the world ill and are on piles of antibiotics or those that have a lot of emotional stress—like the kind that comes from being placed in many homes before they're even six months old—good nutrition is the first place to turn. The same is true for animals with chemical stress (such as getting multiple vaccines in a single visit to the vet or experiencing early worming): the immune system is compromised. Good nutrition is your best bet there too.

Who is qualified to prescribe this? If this is all news to you and you are drawn to try raw food, I have listed several books in the back that are worth exploring—you can qualify yourself to prescribe good nutrition! Many of the authors of these books do consultations as well. Also, there are some great holistic veterinarians who are also well versed and offer consultations.

A cautionary note: you can always find something on the Internet to support your belief. You can also find random people who consider themselves experts on feeding animals. Sometimes the average pet owner uses online sources to become an "expert" on animal nutrition overnight. But if you go that route, you can make some big mistakes. I encourage you not to be impulsive here. Take your time, study the resources I offer in the back of the book—all knowledgeable and trustworthy sources—and find a professional you trust to consult with too.

With regard to prepared foods, if you have one in your area, a holistic pet food store is the best option. Usually the people in these stores are well versed in the best products available. On the other hand, the well-meaning teenager working in a major chain pet store may not be the best person to trust to provide expert advice.

What can I try at home? Real raw food if you can, cooked if that's too much of a stretch, and premium pet food if neither one of the others is going to work for you. Consider supplementing premium pet food with some raw or real food. When vets says "no table scraps," they mean don't feed pizza, bread scraps, or pasta.

I have taught people how to read pet food labels since 1998, and I have a principle you can apply when you're thinking about premium pet foods. The first five ingredients must be actual *food!* That's it. And it's harder to find prepared foods that meet that standard than you might imagine.

Also, before you consider diet, get a baseline of your animal's health, using your own senses. What is the coat like? Is it shiny on the spine and dull on the sides (where the digestive tract is)? What does the animal's breath smell like? Do the ears smell? Assess your companion's level of energy, and get blood work done so you have a medical baseline too.

Homeopathy

Once you've ensured that your animal companions are getting the right nutrition for their species, supporting them at the most fundamental level, you can start working with substances that function on a more vibrational level. Giving homeopathic remedies is an excellent next step.

What is it? Allopathic medicine subscribes to rational thought and focuses on looking at treating disease. Homeopathy shares the commitment to empirical thought, but its focus is on the individual.

Homeopathy is used to treat individuals with emotional upsets as well as physical conditions, and a homeopathic remedy itself also has a "personality" and associated emotions.

Any reputable source of education on homeopathy will take you back to its founder, Samuel Hahnemann, and all the way back to 1796. Yet people forget that Hippocrates played with its basic principle of like curing like. Hahnemann developed the theory even further and based homeopathy on "the law of similars." According to this law, the core essence of the illness or challenge being treated is delivered to the body via a highly diluted homeopathic solution. As the system is exposed to this highly diluted substance, rather than trigger further illness, the substance activates the body's natural system of healing, or homeostasis, which is the state and tendency toward equilibrium, whether metabolically within a cell or in an organism.

It was when Hahnemann discovered that he experienced symptoms from cinchona bark that were similar to the symptoms he experienced when he had malaria that he started to play with the idea that treatments could produce symptoms in a healthy person similar to those of the disease being treated—and the world of homeopathy was born. Homeopathic remedies contain a very small, highly diluted amount of the disease or issue being treated that is added to a tincture and shaken.

Veterinarian Richard Pitcairn considers homeopathy a medical art and believes its elegance as a treatment modality should be much more widely recognized. He describes how homeopathy works in his book *Dr. Pitcairn's Complete Guide to Natural Heath for Dogs & Cats*:

> We know that a bee's sting will cause a certain typical
> reaction, including swelling, fluid accumulation (causing
> a bump), redness of the skin, pain, and soreness.
> Typically, all of this is made worse by the application
> of heat and pressure. Some sensitive individuals also
> experience mental symptoms such as apathy, stupor, and
> listlessness, or the opposite—whining and tearfulness.
> If a homeopathically prepared dilute solution of bee

venom is given to a person with these symptoms, even if
the symptoms are caused by something other than a bee
sting, the condition will begin to improve.[3]

Homeopathy prescribes in two ways. First, there is an acute or constitutional diagnosis, which is something as simple as looking at the
symptoms being presented and giving a common remedy that offers
relief to those symptoms. As Dr. Pitcairn stated, if the symptoms are
the same as a bee sting, apis mellifica (honeybee venom) would be
indicated for this condition.

That's the simplest aspect of homeopathy. In other words, everyone
may respond to poison ivy the same way, so a highly diluted dose of
poison ivy is a simple acute fix for those same symptoms. But then we
look at the emotional layer, it's not as simple. Everyone handles grief differently, for example. Now the right remedy needs further investigation.

Illness shows up in individuals differently because it reflects a
combined pattern of the illness that is unique to that particular individual. Enter the constitutional diagnosis—a much deeper level.
Again, homeopathy addresses the individual rather than the disease,
so the practitioner looks at the whole personality (the constitution)
of the animal, as well as the animal's response to the disease. The
constitution provides a road map leading to the common thread in
the animal's history that relates to the current disease, and following that thread leads to the remedy. There is some experimentation
involved as well. Many remedies may be applied before coming to a
cure. Homeopathy is a process.

As I mentioned earlier, remedies themselves have a personality.
Some remedies may be beneficial for an animal throughout its lifetime
because the animal mirrors the personality of the remedy. At other
times, to put the animal back on track, a single round of that particular remedy would help. For example, an "apis" animal might be fidgety,
restless, irritated, and not like to be left at home alone. It might not
want to be brushed. So, keeping apis on hand might be a good idea
in this case just to ground the animal, even if it hasn't been anywhere
near a bee!

While standard drugs temporarily discontinue the pattern of the disease, there is a good possibility that the disease will return because the disease's neuropathway still exists, so the same pattern can recur. Homeopathy, on the other hand, peels the onion layer by layer until there is no disease pattern left.

Who does this help? Everyone. There is a homeopathic remedy for just about anything, from urinary tract infections to ear mites, from arthritis to grief.

Who is qualified to administer or prescribe this? There are plenty of books available that offer the basics, and you can go into any health food store and pick up a little bottle of a homeopathic remedy. You can certainly educate yourself enough to address acute cases. To truly address a chronic problem, disease, or a behavioral challenge, though, a classically trained homeopath or homeopathic veterinarian is called for. Many of them can work by telephone after you first answer a series of interview questions in writing. I list two veterinarians I recommend for this work along with books on the subject in the resources section.

What can I try at home? It's a great idea to have on hand a little homeopathic first aid kit, along with a few remedies to get your animal through times of physical or emotional upheaval. Some really wonderful things to have on hand include the following:

Apis—bee stings, bites, swelling, irritation

Arnica montana—bruising, soreness, muscle aches and pain

Byronia—musculoskeletal conditions that move, and pain that shifts around (compensation patterns from original injury)

Hypericum (St. John's Wort)—skeletal issues; best known for healing nerves and nerve pain

Ledum—puncture wounds

Nux vomica—vomiting, diarrhea, constipation, colic, bloating

Phosphorus—skin and ears, gingivitis, abscess, cough

Pulsatilla—urinary incontinence, arthritis, and nasal discharge

Rhus tox—arthritis, trouble getting up and moving in the morning, irritated skin

Ruta graveolens—tendons, flexor tendons, joint pain, and injuries

Silicea—vaccinosis, itching, mange, abscess, and decaying teeth

Sulphur—ear mites, fleas, lower immune system, and helps with many chronic diseases

Thuja—vaccinosis, cystitis, corneal ulcers, injuries to the brain and spinal cord

While this list barely scratches the surface of the available remedies, I hope it will whet your appetite for learning more about the powerful alchemy of homeopathy.

There is crossover between remedies and herbal uses as well. Calendula is a great homeopathy remedy and a wonderful herb for healing wounds by means of a compress. Many salves are also calendula based. Chamomile can also be used as a compress, and whether used as an herb or a homeopathic remedy, its effect is calming.

Then there are the remedies that have extra strong personalities. This is worth mentioning because while the above-listed remedies have physical healing abilities, they also have personality attributes that can be matched to an animal. For example, if an animal had a big history of overmedication and its system was compromised, nux vomica would be indicated, but so would pulsitilla. A pulsitilla dog would be more nurturing and loving, though needy. A nux dog would be more sensitive and irritated. The subtle difference of the remedy matched with the animal makes all the difference for immediate healing.

It is worth mentioning some of the remedies with the bigger, more dramatic personalities, which are listed below. See if any of these match the challenges your animal faces at home:

Actonite—a traumatic fear, the first stages of inflammation, cystitis, pacing

Arsenicum—fear of strangers, anxiety, fear of being alone, tendency to hide from new people

Belladonna—intense, hot, aggressive, delirious, fever, hotspots, throbbing

Ignatia—grieving, melancholy, weeping, tummy ache, a sinking feeling

Stranonium—terror that leads to aggression, nervousness, confusion

Two other homeopathic remedies that aren't always found in the classical homeopathic books are melatonin and serotonin. Taken homeopathically, these have no side effects. Melatonin is a hormone released by the pineal gland as the sun goes down; it helps us want to sleep. The homeopathic form can help relax anxiety and has been known to help dogs with a fear of thunder. Serotonin is a neurotransmitter that is known to balance mood, help "even things out," and relieve anxiety.

There are also plenty of homeopathic combinations, sprays, and offshoots. They may be frowned upon by traditional homeopaths, who consider this unethical, but I've seen plenty of them work well.

Finally, homeopathy is known for *nosodes,* or homeopathic vaccines. There is a nosode out there for pretty much everything you would vaccinate your animal for. For example, a nosode vaccination against EPM (a neurological disorder in horses) is produced from the spinal cord of an EPM-positive horse. The parvo nosode is created from the diarrhea of a parvo-infected dog.

You might be asking, "Isn't this the same like-heals-like theory regular vaccines are based on too?" True, vaccines offer a teeny bit of the illness, but the method of delivery is in question. In homeopathy, a flu virus nosode is in a solution of 10 percent alcohol and 90 percent water. Vaccines are made up of the viral or bacterial substance that the vaccine is supposed to prevent, called antigens, plus chemicals to enhance the immune response, called adjuvants and preservatives. The adjuvants can range from aluminum to sodium borate, and the preservative is almost always mercury. You can easily see why this can be hard on the system.

Vaccines are political and personal. Most holistic practitioners warn against the old-school thought of annual vaccines and offer advice on how to build the immune system instead. This is something that is worth investigating on your own, so you can make an informed decision for yourself and your animal family. If you still choose to vaccinate with pharmaceutical vaccines, please consider many of the healing techniques in this book as ways to support the immune system and ease the impacts of the vaccines.

It is hard to argue against science when we know that 300 million people died of smallpox, that the disease has been completely eradicated, and that only two vials of it still exist on this earth. That's impressive, yet excessive vaccination is still prevalent in this country. Research shows that the antibodies in one rabies vaccine usually protect a dog for at least half its life, if not longer, yet some vets vaccinate every year—some states even insist on it.

Don Hamilton, DVM, believes the overvaccination problem today stems from a disease called old dog distemper, something that showed up in older dogs that had only been vaccinated in their youth. At the time, it was perceived that the disease showed up because these dogs hadn't had enough vaccines. Suddenly, more was better when it came to vaccinations. Meanwhile, Dr. Hamilton surmises that the old dog distemper was probably *vaccinosis*—a bad reaction to vaccination.

> ## BE CAREFUL WITH VACCINES
>
> Vaccines should only be given to healthy animals. Also, note the disclaimer and the instructions on vaccines—that they should be administered to a front leg so the leg can be removed if tumors or cancer occur. Please consider the whole of your animal's health when you decide to vaccinate.

Awareness of the downsides of vaccination is developing among traditional Western veterinarians now, and these days it is much easier than it ever was before to have that conscious conversation and to weigh the benefits against the drawbacks. Ultimately, it is your animal companion, and it is your choice. Instead of automatically demanding new vaccinations, more and more doggy day cares, kennels, and barns are taking titers tests to see the amount of antibodies remaining in the system from original vaccinations or nosodes. Horse shows and dog shows are coming to this awareness too.

■ ■ ■

We started this chapter on a very down-to-earth note, discussing the importance of feeding your animals well to support their health and make everything else you do more effective. Then we moved into the subtler world of homeopathic remedies. There's a lot more where that came from! Chapter 9 is all about healing modalities that work on a vibrational level.

9

Vibrational Medicine:
Energy Technologies

The clearest way into the Universe
is through a forest wilderness.
JOHN MUIR

The energy technologies in this chapter are truly vibrational medicine. While they work on a very subtle level, using them could be exactly what's needed to trigger *homeostasis,* which is our goal. We naturally tend toward homeostasis, so when this balanced state is disrupted, the body has ways to return to it, ways to reset. When a major disease or intense stress is present, the reset can be a struggle.

The essential oil of a leaf or the aroma of a flower could be just the influence your animal needs to return to homeostasis. In your energy-healing work with animals, you will be drawn to some of the elements in this chapter more than others. You may find yourself researching every study that's been done on the humble dandelion as an herb, an essence, and more. Or you may just jump in and feel your way to modalities or technologies that could help your animal achieve better health!

You can use all of the technologies in this chapter on their own or in concert with bodywork or energy work to create healing. You can also use them in conjunction with medicines prescribed by the vet and other conventional treatments. Aromatherapy doesn't contraindicate chemotherapy, for example, and in fact, it may be just the thing to relax the system into accepting such an intense treatment.

You have a wonderful natural asset on your side when you work with these vibrational methods: animals don't discriminate about whether energy technologies work. They assimilate them much faster because they aren't burdened with a belief system that questions them, thereby creating resistance to their power. So while all of these methods can work for humans too, our animal companions are naturally open.

As is true of many of the techniques you've learned about so far, vibrational medicine, subtle energies, and energetic technologies depend on intention to work. When we combine a flower essence with the intention of easing grief for our heartbroken dog, the effects can be stunning.

Muscle testing and pendulums are excellent methods to employ when you're trying to decide if you should try one of these technologies. Simply ask questions like these:

Will this modality help me heal this situation?

Will this modality bring my animal into a state of homeostasis?

Once you've received a yes or a no, you can also test for dosage this way:

Should I give five drops?

The beauty of this subtle energy work is that you always have the opportunity to increase your ability to "feel into" the vibration. In the case of a flower essence, crystal, essential oil, or mineral, sometimes all you need to do is hold it in your hand and feel the vibration for a moment, and you will actually glean the ancient wisdom, the DNA, of the technology and know whether it's a match for your animal companion.

TUNING IN TO VIBRATIONAL MEDICINE

Here is a great exercise you can do to develop your ability to feel into the vibrations of a substance you're considering using to help your animal feel better. First, make sure you have a journal handy. Then pick up a crystal, and let it speak to you. Write down what you feel and experience. It may literally speak to you!

Now take your journal and sit with your back to a tree. Listen for what the tree has to tell you and write it down.

Next, sit with an herb, one that is still thriving in the ground or in a pot. Let your hand hover about three inches above the plant and feel for the energy and life force that radiate from it. Jot down your impressions. Then, the next time you purchase an herb in a package, see if you still feel that life force.

All of these exercises will help you fine-tune your sensitivity to energy technologies.

Essential Oils

What are they? Essential oils are the volatile oils extracted from plants. They contain the essence of the plant: therefore, essential oils. Essential oils are at least as old as the Bible, and anointing with oil is a practice that's been used in ceremony for millennia. Embalming methods in ancient Egypt and China also used oil. Today a common way to use essential oils is through aromatherapy, and we use it to alleviate disorders, shift moods, and heal various conditions. Aromatherapy oils can be used topically or inhaled. The important thing to know is that each individual oil has a different purpose. Essential oils are a subtle technology useful for dealing with complex things, yet they are so simple and pure that their effects can be immediate.

An essential oil, consisting of the plant's energy and frequency, is contained in teeny molecules that vaporize easily and can quickly enter the nose and bloodstream. They are thought to affect every cell of the body within twenty minutes and are then metabolized like other nutrients. Because these volatile molecules are so light and move so quickly, they can cross the blood-brain barrier as well as move into tissues and influence cells. You can reach the entire body at once with this treatment method.

The oil itself carries a very high frequency, while mental, physical, and emotional challenges vibrate at lower frequencies. On an energetic and therapeutic level, these potent little molecules can raise an animal's frequency almost immediately.

Essential oils go straight into the limbic system, the brain's overseer of emotion, behavior, long-term memory, and the olfactory system. This is why we can have an emotional response to someone's perfume, and why the aromas of certain things can trigger memories for us, with feelings attached, good or bad.

Essential oils are thought to bring on the immune defense properties of plants by regenerating and oxygenating the system. They are also thought to feed cells and help them retain nutrients. They have proven to be wonderful antioxidants, working as free radicals and preventing mutations. Certain essential oils are known to be antifungal, antibacterial, antiviral and antiseptic, and anti-infectious. They help with detoxification and overall emotional, spiritual, mental, and physical well-being. And as if all that were not enough, aside from their healing properties, essential oils are useful in soaps, cleaning products, incense, and perfumes.

If you're wondering how essential oils can be so powerful, consider pheromones, the "essential oil" chemicals that various animals secrete to elicit a specific response. The chemical involved can have a social, sexual, or emotional function, among others. The social function is about territory. With cats, even those that have been spayed or neutered and can no longer actually spray, they still produce a territorial scent to create a boundary.

Pheromones can also be produced or replicated commercially. A case in point is commercially available cougar pee, used to ward coyotes off farms. And for a more urban or suburban household, we can use scents to ward off the neighbor's tomcat or even to help ease the effects of bringing a new animal into the home.

Case in point: I once worked with a very protective German shepherd named Jake who had been walking around his suburban Chicago property peeing in lines for a week. When his worried owner brought Jake to the vet, a few simple questions ruled out any serious health concern. Then the owner discovered that there were two coyotes in the area. Jake had been warning them with his pee not to set foot on his property—or else!

Who does this help? The answer is anything or anyone who has nostrils and breathes through them! Essential oils can help with anything from being able to breathe more deeply to relaxing to expediting healing after surgery. They also help when it comes to grounding, easing anxiety, elevating depression, and much, much more.

One of the most important things our wonderful autonomic nervous system takes care of for us is breathing. It also takes care of our heartbeat and the blinking of our eyes. But when we humans are faced with something that generates anxiety, such as an equestrian performance—a big jump or a dressage test—our fear can inhibit our breathing. And then, in turn, our limited breath can minimize our horse's ability to breathe deeply and stay relaxed. So while I'm enthusiastic about using essential oils for healing your animals, it's beneficial to your animals when you use them too!

Let's say your dog was attacked years ago, and now every time you walk your dog on a leash, you look around suspiciously in full defense mode in case anyone else is out walking their dog. Or let's say your dog attacked another dog and now has leash aggression—aggressive behavior that only shows up when it's on a leash. For us, these scenarios share a common denominator: we, the humans, forget to breathe. The dog senses this and may hold its breath too. Now we're both anticipating an upcoming disaster.

In other words, we have suspended our own ordinary functioning—normal breathing—because our emotion around an event is bigger than the event itself. For horses and their riders caught up in this kind of anxiety, something as simple as applying some peppermint or eucalyptus on both the horse's and the rider's chests works wonders. It helps both breathe more deeply and relax into the ride. Another good choice is frankincense, as it's good for the lungs and is known to calm and slow breathing.

Cats and certain dog breeds with very short nose canals such as pugs, Boston terriers, and many bulldogs can't use essential oils in the same manner as the rest of the world because there's not enough distance between the nasal canal and brain—the delivery is faster than the speed of light. Giving oils to these animals requires being more selective in how you administer the oils. For instance, you might put the oil on a washcloth near their bed or their food bowl.

A special note about birds: Birds have a very hard time with essential oils, so using them is not at all advised. In fact, many birds have a tough time if their cage is in the kitchen, surrounded with cooking smells and particles, because their respiratory systems are so fragile.

DANGERS IN YOUR HOME

Most of the animals we keep as companions are very sensitive, and their noses are closer to the ground than ours. For this reason, we need to be careful about the cleaning solutions we use in our homes, which can be dangerous for our friends with noses to the floor. Air fresheners are very hazardous—especially the kind you plug into the wall. Not only do the toxic chemicals immediately hit the blood-brain barrier, the barefoot animals in our households also soak them up through their feet. Pesticides are another treacherous form of toxicity for our pets, again entering through nose and feet and penetrating the blood-brain barrier. Be very careful with any substance that has a strong smell in your home.

Who is qualified to do or to prescribe this? There are many online schools and certification programs for aromatherapy and essential oils. There doesn't seem to be a licensing procedure, but there is a National Association for Holistic Aromatherapy. Most people who do this professionally combine it with another practice like massage therapy, animal communication, or a veterinary practice.

The benefit of working with someone who has studied essential oils is that they're as familiar with the properties of the oils as a chef is with the properties of foods. They also know how to combine oils and which oils work better when combined with others.

Can I try this at home? Yes, and when you're working with animals, there is a very simple way to select the oils: the animals themselves get to pick the frequency they need! If an animal doesn't like something, you'll know it right away—it will turn its head away or even walk away. But if it likes it enough to want to eat the oil right out of your hand, you know you're on to something—it's that simple. You won't find an animal on the fence about smells, especially if they bring up negative memories and emotions. Playing like this with essential oils is truly one of the greatest ways to help our animals experience their own innate healing ability.

Please note: if you are pregnant, be careful. Educate yourself about handling essential oils because they are very powerful, and be sure to dilute the oils in vegetable oil.

A Simple Guide to the Oils and Their Four Main Jobs

> Grounding—Bergamot, Cedar, Patchouli, Sandalwood
>
> Calming and Relaxing—Chamomile, Jasmine, Lavender, Sweet Marjoram
>
> Enlivening—Carrot Seed, Citrus, Neroli, Peppermint, Rosemary, Sage
>
> Purification—Fennel, Juniper (for toxin buildup), Lemon, Lime, Myrrh, Tea Tree

While each of these oils offer emotional support, they offer physical help as well.

My Personal Favorites

There are a number of essential oils that I personally love, live with, and work with. Let me run down a few of them:

Carrot seed—clears the head, relieves stress, is good for the liver and skin issues, also helps hooves

Fennel—for lymph, nausea, and curbing appetite

Frankincense—eases muscle pain

Lemon—eases acidity and is good for arthritis and gout

Neroli—helps with tension and calms the nervous system in general

Peppermint—helps headaches, calms digestion and pain, refreshes the spirit, alleviates depression and mental fatigue

Rosemary—for toning muscles, circulatory fatigue, digestion, and detoxing

Tea Tree—antifungal, antibacterial, antiviral

For a more complete list of essential oils and what you can use them for, see the Resources section in this book.

Flower Essences

No matter what you might be worried about in this moment, if you stop and gaze at a flower, your breathing will suddenly change. You can't help but notice its beauty, and it has a frequency that even an energy denier would have to acknowledge. Simply noticing and acknowledging the flower changes your vibration. A flower resonates, a flower glows, and a flower demonstrates that beauty exists. Sometimes a little flower popping through the stark earth after a long winter brings a soft breath of hope. This is what flower essences are all about.

A flower essence is a diluted extract of the perfection and essence of the flower. When you use flower essences, a subtle sense of well-being seems to move through your entire being like a breath. Flower essences just seem to take the edge off. They are similar to herbal remedies, homeopathy, and essential oils in that they are used in a diluted form that then energizes to become more potent than their original form. Flower essences are made by leaving flowers in the sun to extract their essence, then diluting it in water, and then preserving it with alcohol to make "the mother tincture." From there, the remedy is diluted again in spring water to make the solution we will give to our animals or ourselves. Flower essences are mainly used to support the body, mind, and spirit, though sometimes they can completely shift and even help a condition.

In his book *Vibrational Medicine: The #1 Handbook of Subtle-Energy Therapies,* Dr. Richard Gerber introduces us to Dr. Edward Bach, who discovered flower essences. Bach knew there was much more to illness than the physical level of it. As Gerber explains:

> Edward Bach was a pioneering medical thinker who discovered a link between stress, emotions, and illness decades before most contemporary physicians had begun to address the issue. From his initial insight on the emotional contributors to illness, Bach sought to find a simple and natural way to return people to a level of harmonious balance. It was this search for a cure in nature that eventually led Bach to discover the healing properties of homeopathic remedies and ultimately the essences of flowers.[4]

Dr. Bach went on to develop what we've come to know as Bach Flower Remedies. There are now several other companies that create flower essences, some of which dedicate themselves solely to flower essences for pets.

Here is a brief list of some of the challenges flower essences can address:

Challenge	Flower Essence
Unaccountable fears	Aspen
Jealousy of a new animal or baby	Holly
Overattachment to the past	Honeysuckle
Repeating unsuccessful behavior patterns	Chestnut bud
Period of change; new family	Walnut

How might you use these with your animals in practice? Let's say you adopted a new puppy. Adding a little honeysuckle, chestnut bud, and walnut essences to its drinking water would help ensure a smooth transition. You name it; there is a flower essence for it. A single essence, mimulus, works for animals that are afraid of lightning or going to the vet, and those that shake or are timid. When you give this essence to such an animal, it becomes more confident and courageous and can enjoy life without fear.

Some essences are a wonderful support for the entire system and can be used in conjunction with training and just about every healing technique. They're helpful to an animal undergoing chemotherapy and even at the end of the animal's life to support the shift.

Herbs

Herbal medicine is considered both folk and botanical medicine. Countless studies have been done on herbs, and the medical community loves to say that the results are inconclusive. But the fact is many herbs are fundamental to Western pharmacology. And ancient and indigenous cultures have relied solely on the healing and synergistic properties of herbs for hundreds if not thousands of years.

It's said that a plant is only as good as the soil it's grown in. A good pH balance is necessary for the soil to produce balanced growth. Herbs have deep taproots, so the healthier the soil is under the surface, the better; the trace minerals deeper in the soil don't get destroyed the way they do in topsoil. Bottom line: it's important to know the source of your herbs, and keep in mind that organic is always better.

There are a few different herb "worlds." The ones I will be referring to here are mostly American, Native American, and European herbs. Chinese herbs, a cornerstone of Traditional Chinese Medicine, are an entirely different set of herbs, concoctions, and tinctures that requires a very solid education to administer correctly. Another herbal pharmacopeia that I will just mention here are the Ayurvedic herbs from India.

What all of the herbal systems share is the aim of creating balance in the person or animal ingesting them. Some herbal remedies are a single chemical compound extracted from a plant for medicinal purposes, while others are whole-plant preparations referred to as phytomedicine (plant medicine). In Europe, phytomedicine may be prescribed along with drugs. In the United States, we find over-the-counter supplements sold in specialty stores as well as watered-down versions sold in some grocery stores.

In some Native American cultures, herbs are considered both medicinal and spiritual. South American herb lore is magnificent, recognizing the power of plants and the significance of how and where they are grown and using that information accordingly. For example, maca, a Peruvian ginseng, is an herb grown at high altitudes with little oxygen. This means it has to work harder to grow. As a result, it is a strong herb, aerobic in nature, which rewards with lots of energy, longevity, and the stimulation of hormones. This holistic view of the plant is built in to the technology of South American herbal healing.

AN EXPERIMENT WITH HERBS

In the early 1990s, I broke my ankle in a riding accident. I now have a plate and six screws in it. From the very first, right after the doctors put it in a cast, I made myself a drink every morning of pineapple (for the bromelain—good for bone healing), comfrey, horsetail, and parsley, and I took

MSM (a supplement with anti-inflammatory properties that helps soft tissue) and vitamin C. I also placed my hands on the cast over my ankle several times a day, doing yoga and stretching with whatever could and would move. The next time I went in for x-rays, the only way the doctor could find the breaks was by locating the screws in those places. There's testimony to the healing power of herbs and energetic healing!

Hulda Regehr Clark, PhD, was a naturopath who had a theory that all cancer starts with parasites. She launched a full-on attack on cancer using herbal remedies to rid the body of parasites (along with a little zapper that zaps parasites and bacteria). Her book *The Cure for All Cancers,* includes many remedies and tinctures. There is a diluted parsley water recipe along with more common herbal recipes. For cleansing humans of parasites, she recommends a combination of black walnut hulls, wormwood, and common cloves. For animals, herbal cleansing is the safest way to remove parasites; chemical wormers are so toxic that at the end of the day, they create many other challenges.

If you have a weak stomach when it comes to parasites, you may want the CliffsNotes version of Hulda Clark's book! Otherwise, her ideas about cleansing and her recipes are fascinating reading.

Herb Delivery Methods

- Poultices and compresses. Moisten cotton bandages with an herbal tincture or use a compress, either warm or hot, held in place with a bandage. You can also use a tea bag (a chamomile tea bag is a great way to calm the irritation of an insect bite). These methods also work well for injuries.

- Infusions. Make a tea, either using a tea bag or loose roots and flowers steeped in hot water.

- Tinctures. These are the herbs preserved in liquid, usually alcohol. I've also seen herbs preserved in honey, though the shelf life is much shorter. There are also herbal syrups, or serums.

- Salves and ointments. These are wonderful to have on hand for healing wounds (and even preventing wrinkles!). With the right delivery system (the oil used), they can penetrate immediately into the skin.

Animals sometimes wander into the herbs they need, if they have the chance. As horses forage through their grazing day, they frequently find the herb they need. Alfalfa is mistakenly *fed* to horses, though it is a wonderful herb with healing properties. As an equine herb, in really small doses it can detoxify, aid in balancing the hormonal system, and help treat ulcers—yet when fed as a food, alfalfa can create ulcers! So please, ask your vet about your horse.

Working with a practitioner and/or consulting another reliable source is very important because herbs are complex beings that volunteer to help, but if overused, they can be toxic. You know how painful it is to brush up against a nettle leaf, yet in a tea or even a pill form, nettle helps the kidneys and works as an expectorant. It's all in the usage. There are as many disclaimers on several herbs as there are on television commercials for Viagra. So again, be mindful and responsible, and then feel confident that it is safe to treat your animal companion with herbs. I have yet to hear a cat complain about excessive catnip!

Some of My Favorite Herbs

Burdock. Burdock is used as an antioxidant. It helps control cell mutation and detoxifies while aiding the immune system, liver, and gallbladder. It even gets rid of skin disorders. I had a client whose horse fell into an old mine shaft while out on a trail ride. They were able to pull her out and save her, but the cuts on her legs were in such places that they couldn't give stitches. The fear of infection from these open wounds was high. I consulted an herbalist, who told me that burdock root promotes natural stitching of the skin, so I got a coffee grinder and a bag of burdock root and ground the root up very finely. I placed the powder in the most awkwardly placed wounds by blowing it into them, and sure enough, the skin grew back quickly and beautifully! Later when I moved to Florida, this burdock came in very handy as many horses there get what are called "summer sores," insect larvae that find their way into cuts and cause awful sores. Burdock has saved several clients' horses again and again!

Milk Thistle. Hands down, this is my go-to herb to clean the liver and promote new cell growth in the liver. In Chinese medicine, the eyes are related to the liver, so milk thistle is a subtle support for the eyes, in addition to other remedies. It also helps gallbladder function, the adrenals, and the immune system. The other organ associated with the liver is the skin, the biggest and most exposed organ of all. Milk thistle taken internally is a wonderful way to help the skin from the inside out (along with lots of digestive support).

Calendula. This herb is usually used topically and is good for the skin. It helps with irritation and is very soothing. Calendula and comfrey are almost always found in any sort of wound-healing salve, and they make a safe, nontoxic potion for skin disorders. Calendula is very comforting in any area that has had to be shaved.

Turmeric. If there is one thing that is being touted as an anticancer herb and natural antibiotic, it's turmeric. It fights free radicals and protects the liver, and of course turmeric has been used as a spice in curries for years. You must watch the dosage, though, because it can be hard on the stomach. It remains a wonderful anti-inflammatory—great to add to an older dog's diet!

Eyebright. You can use this as an eye wash. It is great for aging animals that are starting to get cataracts. If you're going to apply it to the eyes, make sure you buy an eye wash, though, as opposed to the tincture! The tincture is very good taken internally; I've seen a lot of positive changes with it.

Eucalyptus. This is great for respiratory challenges; it reduces swelling and increases blood flow.

Crystals and Gemstones

Our darling planet Earth is 4.6 billion years old—and she looks fabulous! We know her age from radiometric dating, which measures the rate of decay in minerals. Even decay is a form of vibration, and this illustrates the dynamic nature of rocks, crystals, and even dirt—always vibrating. The level and frequency of these vibrations are what we can glean from them and use in energy healing. In other words, crystals are as old as dirt! Crystals actually are dirt—call them fancy dirt.

Using crystals for healing is an ancient technology—so prevalent, in fact, that it's part of our language and associated with both spirituality and royalty. For example, we aim to make it to "the pearly gates," or we hope to see "the crown jewels." We have found jade in Egyptian tombs, thought to guide souls in the afterworld. The Chinese use jade to this day for healing. Gemstones and semiprecious stones are sought after and actually considered a sign of wealth. The good news for the rest of us is that all of this "ancient dirt" is magical earth medicine.

The word "crystal" is derived from the Greek word *krustallos,* which means both ice and rock crystal. "Quartz" means a clear, colorless mineral. Crystals are also used as electronic components. Salt, glass, and jewelry are all associated with crystals as well.

Crystals are formed in the earth and are often found combined with other minerals. There are several steps in the crystallization process, in which elements combine to create heat; the crystal is formed in the cooling process. Other shifts can occur through exposure to or pressure from liquids, solids, and temperature. While they seem to be a solid form, crystals are still expanding, shifting, and mutable. Perhaps these qualities are what we seek from them.

Wearing gemstones in necklaces to feel pretty or putting a lucky stone in your pocket for a job interview automatically lifts your frequency. Did you know that this is no different from using crystals for healing? Knowing that a particular crystal has a wonderful purpose or healing quality, coupled with your need and/or intention, ups the ante a bit. Why not enjoy this wonderful magic?

You can attach crystals to a dog's or a cat's collar, or you can put it next to their bed. Just be careful your pet doesn't eat the crystal! If you ride horses, you can wear the crystal while riding or attach it to the halter or saddle pad. You can hold one with you as you work to improve your telepathic abilities and communicate with your animal. Crystals hold energy, memory, and even technology.

You can use crystals to mitigate emotions and behaviors in your animals, such as possessiveness, clinginess, separation anxiety, grief, demands, lack of confidence, and even the need to reboot their polarity. Many use crystals to bring animals back into their body. Crystals can help to amplify good behavior, improve communication, and promote well-being. Crystals can be used to treat physical symptoms as well, such as inflammation, migraines, muscle soreness, and backaches. They're helpful post surgery and for system balancing too.

If you brought a new family member into the household and they're not getting along with everyone, one option is to set up a crystal grid. You can use peridot and tiger's eye for jealousy, rose quartz for emotional balance, and citrine for self-esteem. Place these various crystals around the room with the intention of creating greater harmony.

If you and your animal companions have lost a member of the family and you all tend to sleep in your room, setting up a crystal grid to surround all of you would be a great way to heal the grief. With grief, you want to allow everyone's feelings to come and go like ocean waves. You also want a sense of being able to let go and allow an animal to feel at peace while everyone is processing, each in their own way. Perhaps your animal has lost its leader or cohort. Calcite helps such an animal feel nurtured, and malachite can uncover any issues surrounding the healing, all the while allowing others in the household to heal as well. It helps to acknowledge and release these emotions instead of burying them. A black obsidian called Apache tears protects even as it allows tears to release, which is very important for grieving. Lapis will help counter any fear and anger—some of the emotions associated with grief that can take us by surprise.

If you're bringing in a new family member with a fear of abandonment, you might try watermelon tourmaline for self-love and well-being, while rose quartz will help with heart healing and tranquility. Add calcite to support the change.

When healing a horse, you can place crystals around the stall or around the horse while you're grooming. For a dog, you can leave them placed around a crate while you are at work, and for a cat, try the favorite sleeping spot. For a bird, place them around the cage.

AMETHYST POWER

When I moved to the farm where I previously lived, the barn had seen two cases of cancer in horses—both of which had happened long before I arrived, though I knew both of the horses. These diseases were of two different types, and they involved two very different horses. The stalls, however, were directly across from each other. It also seemed that the horses in these two stalls had an unusual number of episodes of lameness. I got a few small bags and filled them with amethyst (for calming, healing, and protection) and hung them high in the barn aisle so they wouldn't necessarily be seen. There weren't too many more incidents with the horses inhabiting those stalls.

The one thing that I did notice when I thought about the cancer cases was that there were fluorescent lights hanging in the middle of that particular barn aisle. That end of the barn was the side where hay was loaded into the hayloft, and if the hay loaders didn't remove the fluorescent lights before they got to work, they frequently hit those fixtures, which caused some of the lights to pop out of the socket and shatter (always horrible in a barn). No one knew there was cancer-causing mercury floating around those horses' stalls as a result. Even though the lights broke again and I never did find the mercury, my animals are still alive and have no health issues. I believe the amethyst played a part in protecting them.

Want a booster shot here? Add intention, homeopathy, flower essences, essential oils, and good food to enhance the crystals' ability to shift the energy for your animal companion. Try these modalities until you find what helps your animal.

Sound

One of the most amazing ways to shift energy for us humans is through music. Whether we get all riled up and play air guitar or sing along at the top of our lungs with Bruce Springsteen in the car, sound can transform the moment. Jazz can inspire, classical music stimulates brain function while also calming us physiologically and psychologically, and rock music gives us a jolt of energy. All of this is actually measureable. More and more people in the medical community are integrating music, sound, chanting, bells, drumming, and singing bowls into their practices. Humans scheduled for an MRI are told to choose soothing music for the experience. Crystal singing bowls are known to bring positive effects to the endocrine, autonomic, and immune systems. Of course, all of this magical work also benefits animals!

Music penetrates to the core, which is why sound has been used for centuries in healing and in spiritual ceremonies. People bond over music. Music brings together mathematics, lyrics, and artistry. Music and sound are used for healing and meditation. Why? Sound can change your state immediately because music bridges the left and right brains.

The body as a whole and all its different parts—the cells, tissues, muscles, bones, brain, and emotions—resonate at a certain frequency. Any accident, upset, or illness can throw off the natural rhythm. Things like tuning forks, chanting, drums, Tibetan bowls, didgeridoos, even a deep "Om" (the often-chanted sacred syllable) can restore alignment to the system. Not only does the physical body have a frequency that needs to be tuned up, the chakras and the aura also have their own frequency, which can be in need of a recharge.

Gospel music carries such purity and a heartfelt plea. It can be reflective or uplifting. Hymns, which are prayers set to music, can bring harmony. "Hallelujah" said in unison or sung in song holds a charge because of the ancient wisdom it carries. "Om" also taps into ancient technologies to create union. When they resonate from deep breaths, these ancient prayers and chants carry true healing wisdom, along with the intention brought to their use. Native Americans facilitate this with their healing prayers, music, drums, and song. It is said that singing your prayers gets the message to the angels that much faster. The good news is that animals definitely respond to this modality.

Acutonics is a wonderful emerging healing technique that combines the use of modern tuning forks with the acupuncture meridians. This technique can be used for neurological testing and to scan the body for fractures. It offers a precise, noninvasive approach to healing that benefits the horse, dog, or cat that just doesn't like acupuncture. Like acupuncture, Acutonics helps restore the body to its natural rhythm.

Healing Machines

At some point, we will realize that we created the machines I'm about to present because we had the intention to heal with frequency—and that this is something we can do naturally with our own hands and with all the energetic healing techniques we've discussed so far. Maybe when that light bulb goes on, more of us will be inclined to turn to these natural techniques. Until then, let's acknowledge that it's easier for some people to accept a miracle from a machine than from a healer's hands, essential oils, or herbs. And some of the machines we've created are useful, so let's take advantage of this healing option too.

The Rife Machine, or frequency generator, is a wonderful tool to raise the frequency in a person or an animal. It is based on the work of Royal Rife, who believed that everyone had an electromagnetic "signature," or oscillating blueprint. He reasoned that the underlying causes of illness—parasites, bacteria, viruses, and even yeast (candida)—correspond to specific frequencies. Intensifying that frequency and projecting it at the problem, like a powerful high musical note, could shatter the underlying frequency like glass. Rife created hundreds of frequencies for healing, and I have seen the Rife Machine work on everything from laminitis in a horse to lung cancer in a cat. I've seen it help get the nerves in the hind end of a dog moving again too.

Another modality is I-Therm, which is based on hyperthermia. An ancient Greek physician named Parmenides said, "Give me a chance to create a fever, and I can cure anything." Like the Rife Machine, which only uses heat, I-Therm raises the frequency and the temperature of the blood, and the disease can't exist in that "fever." The Rife Machine has been proven over and over again to yield positive results with diabetes, cancer, and certain injuries. It can locate and specialize, directing blood flow to the affected area. Issues like injuries and nerve disturbances don't stand a chance against this level of heat, circulation, and oxygenation.

The Acuscope (the Electro-Acuscope or Myoscope therapy system) is an awesome machine for injuries. One of the things I love about it is that it can measure the before and after of the injury and give you readings around the body. You can measure the challenge, treat it, and measure again. This is really helpful because you can see how far you have left to go. Sometimes an animal will feel so much better after a treatment that it will reinjure itself, so you have to contain them when you use this machine. But the machine even helps with that by measuring your progress, so you know when to limit the animal's activity.

The Myoscope, a companion instrument to the Acuscope, gently stimulates the muscles, tendons, and ligaments, reducing spasm and inflammation and strengthening tissues damaged by traumatic injury.

And then there is Transcutaneous Electrical Nerve Stimulation (TENS), an instrument that uses electricity to reduce pain by stimulating the nervous system of the body without puncturing the skin in any way.

EXPERIMENTING WITH THE ACUSCOPE

A friend of mine, Allison Waldman, and I did many experiments with her Acuscope machine and even got some great press coverage in Wellington, Florida. I connected with various horses, did a physical scan, and the machine backed up everything I found. In other words, the machine is a pet psychic's dream! We were able to treat a lot of horses and dogs by combining the two methods.

Lasers are probably familiar to you. In healing work they are usually multifrequency, pulsed-light machines that pinpoint soft tissue damage and swelling while helping with circulation and inflammation. Recently, a client told me that a foal of hers had been injured at only weeks old. The mother got stuck lying down in her stall, and in her struggle to get up, she kicked the foal in the head. My client got the baby to the hospital, where they examined the injury on the right side of his head, between his ear and his eye. Sadly, when he moved, it was always to the left, and my client was told that there was no hope of the foal straightening out because of the severe neurological damage to the head. The vets were suggesting they put him down immediately.

My client opted for laser treatment instead (although vets told her she was crazy). When I connected with the foal, I could tell the swelling went further back than had been thought, so I suggested she start treating the top of the head, not just the injury, with the laser. I also suggested that she massage the hind end (to bring the energy all the way back as opposed to its pooling in the head).

After several days, the foal straightened out—literally. He's home now, perfectly normal, and running around. Of course, his name is Magnum, the name of the brand of the laser that helped him!

Exercise

Exercise is a vibrational technology? Take a brisk walk in the park or around the block and see what you think! If you were to scientifically prove to me that there was absolutely zero benefit in my jumping rope three days a week and hiking three to four days a week, I would still do it. Why? Simply because of how I feel when I'm through. I enjoy the endorphins, the relaxation, and taking my mind off stuff. I also know it balances my digestion, my hormones, and my cardiovascular system, and it makes me breathe deeply. I can feel my entire body vibrate with health. These benefits are the same for everyone—and of course for animals. Well-known dog whisperer Cesar Milan says that the order of business is exercise, obedience, and then affection.

When cats feel better, their digestion and mood improve, and it's the same for dogs. Horses in the wild move many miles a day. Geriatric animals do better if they move every day. We all have to move it and shake it every now and then. You know what happens to seniors who sit in the La-Z-Boy recliner—they decline. The same goes for animals.

Building exercise into the day is important, and it can be part of your obedience training too. You can create structured play where you bond and connect while they learn and release endorphins. In the end, you are both contributing to the feel-good blue-ribbon emotions!

Believe it or not, this sort of structured playtime with a cat is quite healthy too. A client recently told me that her one-year-old cat had been attacking her thirteen-year-old cat, but this stopped immediately when she took the one-year-old to a therapeutic swimming facility to get some exercise. Even cats get pent-up emotion and frenetic energy, and it can easily be released through daily exercise.

Exercise alone could be the added component to your overall energy-healing plan that shifts your animal's wellness and behavior. It works quickly, and as long as the animal is physically able to do it, it's worth a try.

NAET

Nambudripad's Allergy Elimination Technique, or NAET, is a method developed by Devi Nambudripad, an acupuncturist. She created a system of clearing allergies by exposing the patient to the allergen and tapping along the related meridian to clear it. So NAET is a combination of acupuncture, kinesiology, and contact with the allergen. Practitioners of NAET keep nearly every substance you can think of in little vials to hold up to the patient for diagnosis. My friend Dr. Roger Valentine, a holistic vet in Los Angeles, even does this remotely just by thinking of the allergen with the animal's person on the phone and working through the meridians. When it works, it appears to be a miracle. He has even cleared up some of my allergy issues!

Magnets

A chapter on energetic technologies wouldn't be complete without at least mentioning magnets. Baylor College of Medicine has proven that magnetic therapies can reduce pain. It's a wonderful technology. Magnets improve blood flow in the tissue while rebalancing the electromagnetic energy of a person or an animal.

Magnets have positive and negative ions, which is how they balance. When you have an injury or an immune challenge, you have an imbalance. As far as the immune system goes, you want to project more negative ions to balance out the system. This is what you can do with magnets, which have healed a great many conditions and are thought to have been used for healing since ancient Egypt. Magnets can help challenges such as hormonal imbalance, pain, inflammation, and even depression.

Unfortunately, many of the available products that use magnets—like horse blankets and dog beds—don't always use them properly. The magnets are balanced incorrectly, so the animal receives both negative and positive ions all at the same time, which is a mixed message. The best way to use magnetic therapy is in short doses and with an expert doing the work.

I had much success with magnets when I was transitioning my thoroughbred from shoes to barefoot. I taped on magnets for a few hours at a time to increase the circulation in his feet, putting them on for a couple of hours and taking them off for a couple over the course of a few days, until he wasn't sore at all.

MAGNETS AT THE READY

Magnets are quite easy to use. I cut magnetic sole inserts (made for humans) into thin strips and keep them in the barn for a quick charge of circulation. I can also use them in leg wraps, on the horse's back, taped to the feet, and in many other ways. My dog can chew most of the above off pretty quickly though. I always figure she got just the voltage she needed!

10

A Few More Important
Energy-Healing Techniques

If animals could speak, the dog would be a blundering
outspoken fellow; but the cat would have the rare grace
of never saying a word too much.

MARK TWAIN

The following energy-healing techniques were actually developed for humans. Although we humans have the advantage of being able to describe the healing or the feelings associated with these techniques, the techniques actually work faster when performed on animals. As I mentioned earlier, animals don't have a belief system about whether the techniques work to get in the way. All of these techniques create relaxation, and the beauty of them is that this happens whether you perform the technique perfectly or not; as with most of the techniques in this book, the important thing is your intention.

Relaxation is a basic requirement to stimulate healing, calm anxiety, and focus performance. When the body is relaxed and out of fight-or-flight mode, healing is a natural response. Illness and nervous behaviors put the system on edge, and when the system is on edge, challenges will continue.

A couple of other things to note before we get started. None of these techniques can hurt an animal. They can all be done remotely if you can't be present for hands-on work. All of them can be taught to pet owners, and while it's best to learn from a qualified practitioner at first, the best way to perfect these techniques is to practice them on your animal companion. None of these methods should be used in lieu of veterinary care or help from a professional animal trainer or behaviorist, but you can use them in addition to further support your animal. In case of an emergency, always get medical attention. Then you can use these techniques to help with healing.

The Scalar Wave

Dr. Valerie Hunt, a former UCLA professor and a pioneer in the science of human energy fields and electromagnetic energy, developed the Bioscalar Wave Technique. UCLA asked Dr. Hunt to study the human aura. At that point she didn't believe such a thing existed but found it an entertaining request and decided to humor the school. Dr. Hunt embarked on a series of experiments and was surprised to discover the presence of an electromagnetic field of energy around the body. To conduct her studies, she brought in Rosalyn Bruyere, an energy healer who wrote *Wheels of Light*, a groundbreaking book on the chakra system, and Emilie Conrad, a dancer who created a system of movement called Continuum.

Her discoveries sparked a spiritual awakening for Dr. Hunt, forcing her to take a hiatus from UCLA. From there she went on to study psychic surgeons in the Philippines and was struck by the laser sharpness, the crystal clarity, with which the surgeons worked. She was in awe of the fact that through intention they could cut through skin, tissue, and bone to get to the negative energy and pull it out—all despite the fact that there were no incisions.

Hunt realized that with single-minded focus, the surgeons were using a standing wave of energy to cut through matter. From there she experimented with various techniques to replicate what they were doing and came up with the Bioscalar Wave—which I call the Scalar Wave for short and is also referred to as a standing wave. She discovered that disease has a chaotic pattern in an incoherent field and that homeostasis has a different pattern, dubbed a pattern of wellness. Chaos cannot exist in the presence of a standing wave of energy; therefore, the standing wave offers an opportunity to reset homeostasis.

After trying different healing methodologies myself, I was introduced to this technique in 1998 and started using it for my own healing. Then I used it with my animals. A couple of years later, with a lot of successful healing under my belt, I started teaching it as a technique to use with animals.

Some of the conditions and illnesses I have successfully treated with this technique include:

- A dog with kidney disease
- A cat with lung cancer
- A student who told me she stopped having weekly migraines
- A cat that was not waking after surgery and didn't look like it was going to make it
- Lameness in dogs, cats, and horses
- Diabetes in dogs and cats—cases too numerous to count
- An aggressive dog—three sessions effected a shift
- Several different horses with pneumonia
- Failed immune systems in dogs, cats, and horses
- Horses with colic
- Dogs with bloat

The list goes on. After a horse trainer in Wellington, Florida, took the class, he did the Scalar Wave on himself and on every horse he rode in competition; he won everything that year.

I do this technique daily, whether for just a moment several times a day or sitting down and spending the time to really go through my entire physical, emotional, and mental systems before I meditate. I do it the minute I sit down in an airplane because I know that flying fast across the country or around the world depletes the aura. Between that and drinking lots of water, I rarely have jet lag.

The Bioscalar Wave is not something that requires a lot of preparation. You don't need a sacred space because you are creating one within your body or the body of your animal companion. It is a go-to technique for me, guaranteed to relax the system, and it can be performed in person or remotely.

Reiki

Reiki is an energetic technique that was developed in Japan in the early 1920s. *Rei* roughly translates to mysterious and *ki* means energy. The technique involves the transference and channeling of universal energy through the palms of the hands and, like all healing work, is done through intention.

There are three skill levels or degrees of Reiki: first, second, and Reiki master. Mikao Usui developed the technique while he was taking a twenty-one-day Buddhist training course involving meditation, fasting, and chanting. He mysteriously awoke to the concept that universal energy could travel from the crown chakra and with focused intention be broadcast through the hands to a recipient.

Usui taught nearly two thousand people how to do Reiki and trained several Reiki masters. A woman named Hawayo Takata brought the work to the United States and attuned several Reiki masters. She also insisted in the 1980s that Reiki masters be paid for their work.

Takata is believed to have Westernized the work as well. While Usui believed hand placement during treatment was intuitive, Takata created a system for hand placement as part of formalizing its usage. More and more, Reiki has been used for specific ailments and injuries.

Though you can use hand placements, this work can be performed remotely. It can be used for self-healing and healing others, including your animals. The flow of energy involved in Reiki healing is inexhaustible. The energy knows where to flow, and this is invaluable for both human and animal.

Theta Healing

Theta Healing, a combination of prayer, thought, and meditation, was created by Vianna Stibal. When the practitioner gets into a meditative state, reaches the theta state, and connects with the Creator, they can move or direct energy. The practitioner doesn't actually do the work by getting into this state but allows the Creator to instantaneously heal on a physical, emotional, and spiritual level.

Stibal was a naturopath, massage therapist, and intuitive reader who was a mother of three children when she discovered she had cancer. Using her style of intuitive readings to heal, she cured herself of the disease. While in a meditative state, she realized that forming a true connection with the Creator helped her shift thoughts, beliefs, and feelings about illness. She started using this technique on others and discovered even more miracles occurring. She became curious about how it was actually working and hired a physicist who used a machine to measure waves of energy. That was how she discovered that she is in the theta state when the connection and healing take place.

EFT: Emotional Freedom Techniques

EFT is a healing method that quiets the nervous system, spurs emotional healing, helps alleviate physical pain, and lessens performance anxiety. The technique involves tapping with the fingers on the meridian system of the body. In Traditional Chinese Medicine, each meridian is associated with an emotion, so with EFT, tapping on a series of points on a meridian mitigates overwhelming feelings and emotions.

Let's go back to a discussion early in the book about the energy and behavior of the animals in your home. As you'll recall, animals naturally come in and out of feelings more fluidly than we do. Sometimes they can get stuck in those feelings and the resultant behaviors because we pile on *our* feelings about their situation—they may not want to continue a pattern or behavior but they're trapped by us. Tapping is an excellent way for us to address our own feelings about an animal's emotional state and to help heal the whole household.

There are three ways we can tap to heal an animal's behavioral or health challenges:

- Tapping on ourselves on behalf of the animal, acting as a surrogate

- Tapping on the animal in the same general area as we would a human, thus activating or deactivating the meridians and the associated organs

- Tapping on both ourselves and our animals

When you tap on your more emotional points, you can do it pretty vigorously. When you do it on your animals, though, you need to be mindful of their degree of sensitivity. Many seeming behavioral issues are actually the result of a head injury, so being delicate is important—and it's still powerful.

EFT can be a challenge with cats because they can easily turn around with a big old swat, claws out, to say, "Yeah, tap this!" Also, in both cats and dogs with short noses (such as pugs and Boston terriers), there may not be space to work with some of the tapping points. (I can do it on my cats, but they are pretty used to me doing weird things to them!) If tapping on a cat's face is too threatening or irritating for them, tapping is still very calming, so you can use your intention and simply tap along the bladder meridian that runs along the back on either side of the spine. The Bladder Meridian, as you have learned, contains points associated with each of the organs and the other meridians, so you can easily calm or stimulate a lot of the same issues you would by tapping on the specific EFT points of the face.

If you do this technique on animals in a shelter, remember how super sensitive and highly stimulated they are. This is an excellent technique for calming, but I like to err on the side of safety for all. That said, the points around the eye are very calming.

The Tapping Points

For the exact points to use, consult an animal acupressure chart. The specific points are not necessarily the same as for humans.

- Inside of the eye: Bladder 1— good for eye and nasal disorders and calms the nervous system

- Outside of the eye: Triple Heater 23—relieves pain

- Under the eye: Stomach 1—any issues with the face, teeth, jaws, or eyes

- Under the nose: Large Intestine 20—nasal challenges, allergies

- Under the lips: Conception Vessel 20—helps relieve fear and anxiety and any issues in the mouth

- Collarbone: Pericardium 1— calms the respiratory system and heart. Remember that on a smaller dog or cat, you are going to be tapping on a lot of other acupressure points as well just because of their size. Kidney 27 is right around there, as is Lung 1. All these points seem to have the focus of better breathing and calming. On a horse you can tap broadly, starting at the P1 point and moving across the chest. Lung 1 is also associated with relieving grief, and Kidney 27 is like the foreman or the boss of all of the organs.

- Top of the head: tapping here you're on the Governing Vessel, known to relieve neck and back pain. It also stimulates the immune system and calms the nervous system. When we tap on ourselves, we generally tap on the top of the head. On a dog or a cat, you can tap there and then broadly tap back down the neck a teeny bit, to where the occipital bone (skull) meets the atlas and axis (top of the neck); this will give the benefits of connecting with Bladder 10, which helps depression and fear. By tapping farther down, you also tap Gallbladder 20 to help nourish the brain and alleviate head and neck tension. On a horse, these points are all right on the top of the head in the area known as the poll.

One of the trickier aspects to tapping on animals is whether they will sit still for it! Horses are inclined to stand still while you do it because they are used to being tied up. But cats have no reason to sit there if they don't want to. Dogs will accept it, but if you are trying to calm down a puppy, beware that your hand may become a toy.

Tapping on ourselves with regard to what's going on with our animals can be very powerful. Through one round of tapping on the issue, you can discover other pieces of the dilemma that hadn't occurred to you before. This is fodder for another round of tapping! If the animal isn't getting better or its behavior isn't shifting, this is a good time to tap on yourself and see what comes up for you.

Once I worked on a horse that had a chronic lameness. His owner and I changed the horse's diet and took off his shoes. I was doing regular sessions of Bioscalar Wave, and we were also using some essential oils. So what was standing in the way of the full recovery we expected? We discovered by tapping on the horse's owner that she was used to having the story of her lame horse to tell. When she quit telling it, the horse got better.

Sometimes people have serious guilt attached to an animal's illness. They may feel sad about it. They may be mad at the vet for not treating the animal properly or for being cold when delivering a diagnosis that was hard to hear. We have a lot of feelings around our animals when they're not well, and tapping is a great way to alleviate these feelings.

Here are some of the issues I have tapped with people and animals:

- Fighting bunnies
- A cat that had been recently adopted and was not fitting into the household
- A dog that wouldn't heal
- A cat with cancer
- A horse that was angry at ponies

- A polo horse that was spooking at the goal
- A horse that had been retired and didn't have a job
- A horse that was grieving the loss of her foal
- A horse that didn't know what his job was and was nervous all the time
- A puppy with separation anxiety
- A dog that hadn't accepted the children in the household

Reconnective Therapy

Eric Pearl was a successful chiropractor who accidentally discovered that the healings that were taking place in his practice were much more powerful than the average bone-moving chiropractic adjustment could account for. Just being close to his hands was healing a great many people. Pearl discovered that he had very high frequencies running through his physical, emotional, and mental systems, and he set about deliberately accessing these and then teaching others. The result was Reconnective Therapy, which claims to transcend energy healing because it doesn't require any complex rituals or techniques. Anyone can learn it.

Other Techniques to Explore

There are many other techniques used on people that could also be applied to animals, and if you're interested in expanding your options, you can dig in and do some research on these:

- Matrix Energetics is a consciousness technology based in physics.

- Access Consciousness is a type of healing that involves changing the consciousness.

- Joe Dispenza teaches a type of healing to shift consciousness.

- Rhys Thomas has an energy medicine school to shift consciousness and access deep healing through transformation.

- The Sylvan Mind Method is also about shifting the consciousness.

- BodyTalk is a healing system that harmonizes the mind-body and uses tapping on the body to normalize energy patterns.

■ ■ ■

Note that these techniques share some words in common: consciousness, access, and transformation. Energy healing recognizes the need for this holistic approach. An illness isn't just an illness, for us or our animals; it is a calling to a deeper healing. When we humans go for a healing session ourselves, we automatically improve the frequency of the entire household.

■ ■ ■

There are plenty of other things we humans can do to set the household thermostat to harmony and help change our animals' energy states. I'll start sharing those ideas next.

11

Using Your Human Superpowers: Creative Tools That You Can Use

Some people talk to animals. Not many listen though.
That's the problem.

A. A. MILNE

If emotion is energy in motion, what's the best thing you can do to shift the emotional energy in your multispecies household? You can work your side of the street, and that's what this chapter is all about. It contains creative tools you can use yourself that can have huge positive impacts on your animal friends. And for all of these, you get to trot out the human superpowers of logic and reason. You're great at thinking—in fact, you're excellent at it! The tools in this chapter are all about changing things, making plans, and putting systems in place—activities natural to your already busy human mind.

Beliefs, Thoughts, Emotions, and Words

The profession of animal communication utilizes the tool of telepathy: the transference of pictures, words, and feelings. This is how we communicated when we were first born, and it's still part of our communication, but after we learned to use language, most of us stopped relying on it much. You could say we've lost tone in our telepathic muscles. In fact, I tell people in my weekend workshops that they may be tired by the end of it because they'll be using a muscle they haven't used in a long time. As with developing any skill or muscle, the key is repetition—practice.

Animals in the wild use telepathy to communicate, and they do so by tracking the lead animal's thoughts, feelings, and body language. Now your *living room* is their wild. When your animals are tracking you, what are they finding out?

Our human minds are all over the map. Within a split second, we can be thinking about what's for dinner, planning a dog hike for the next day, and remembering that we forgot to return our aunt's call. We also get into mental loops—thinking the exact same thoughts over and over again. These can create emotions in us that wind up being unsettling for our animal companions.

You might worry about not calling your aunt back. Or maybe you're frustrated that the day seemed to get away from you. On and on it goes, your thoughts leading to emotions that lower the frequency in your household. Next thing you know, your animals are responding to that drop.

Our beliefs about a situation can actually support a behavior or an outcome that we don't want. For example, I visited a barn a few years back to communicate with a horse. While I was standing in the stall preparing to connect with the horse, her owner repeatedly told me about all the behaviors she didn't like in her horse.

After I communicated with the horse, and before I shared what the horse had to say, I asked the woman how long she had been married. Six months, she told me. I asked her how she would feel if she went to dinner with her new husband to meet his old friends, and he introduced her like this: "She had a terrible upbringing. She drank too much through college, but I think she'll behave tonight." She looked at me dumbfounded for a minute, until I explained that she trotted out these stories about her horse as if she expected the horse to repeat that behavior. And worse, she was telling them right in front of the horse, as if daring her to follow through!

Every time we rehash an old, unhappy story about an animal's behavior, we compound the situation. We're saying we don't expect the animal to do anything else. Soon enough, the animal is piled so high with this baggage that it can barely fit through the door.

I call this the Law of Expectation. When I adopted my horse Rollie, I was told that he didn't like to load into a trailer. This is rather common, but he put up a most excellent fight. Not only did I buy this story about him, I also participated in it. I would go to the barn hours before my riding lesson, have the fight, and eventually get him in the trailer. I expected it. I set my schedule around it! And he never let me down. When I changed my thinking about the situation and expected him to do the *right* thing, guess what? He did a lot better. I have moved him from Seattle to Denver to Florida and back to Seattle without much incident. I had to do some work around this on my end, but I can now put him in a trailer just fine.

One more thing about the words we use around our animals. When we say what we mean and mean what we say, we are very clear. When we say what we're thinking out loud, our mind can't do two things at once: when we say "Sit," we really mean it. I talk out loud to my animals a lot. I don't *try* to send telepathic messages to them (unless I'm out of town). Because the mind thinks in pictures, I automatically send my animals a picture the moment I speak.

Creative Tools

In my first book, *Communication with All Life: Revelations of an Animal Communicator,* I offered some creative tools for helping your animal when it's facing a behavioral or health challenge. These are all things you can do to shift the energy of the household. I have since added to my repertoire and would like to share the full list with you now.

Top Ten

Make a list of the top ten ways your animal is excellent and your best friend (even if you don't believe it this minute!). This is something

I ask my clients to do. For example, let's say you have a shy cat. If you were to list the top ten ways this cat is a hero, you can expect a shift in its behavior. This is also great for people who are upset with their animals. It puts the relationship in perspective and accentuates the positive.

Hierarchy

This one's great for a household that is out of balance, meaning that perhaps one of the dogs or even a cat is running the show. If you were to make a list of the characters in the household (the humans and the animals) that reflects who arrived in the household first, it would put the whole situation into perspective:

- Mom and Dad
- Daughter Maria
- Dog Buffy

Place this list in key spots at home and at work where you're sure to see it. It works subliminally on you and the other humans, and you'll be surprised how much it can shift the household.

Change the Animal's Name

As simplistic as this sounds, I've found the results of doing this are almost too good to be true. By changing the animal's name, you can change their whole persona. If you named your dog Thor and he's biting the neighbor, it might be time to give him a softer and gentler name, like Sammy. Many animals are given tough-guy names, and then people wonder why they're aggressive. Conversely, shy animals often have small names. A student of mine renamed her shy feral cat Panther. And she would say it like this: *Paaanthah!* He came around pretty quickly!

Affirmations

When we affirm the outcome we want rather than obsess about the behavior we don't want, we have a chance to effect a change. One of my dogs came to me so shy and timid that she was basically feral: she'd turn into Stephen King's Cujo whenever she saw a person or an animal approach. When I conduct weekend workshops at my farm, people keep their horses with me, so I can't have that kind of behavior going on in any way, shape, or form. And first and foremost, I didn't want my dog to be trapped in that kind of behavior. I certainly wouldn't be hostage to it.

So here's what I did. Whenever someone drove up to the farm or we saw another dog while we were on a hike, I'd get a singsong voice going and say, "Oh look, it's a friend! We love our friends! We love to make new friends!" Whenever I noticed that there were some people around us that she tolerated, I instantly deemed them friends and used the exact same tone of voice for strangers coming to a workshop. This dog is now *the greeter* for my classes and has a ton of friends, of all species.

Calendars

A calendar can be a very calming tool for an animal that's unsure of what's going on with its busy people, particularly if they go out of town a lot. When appointments and trips are written on a calendar and referred to by a house sitter or caretaker, this has a way of working on the animal that is practically magic.

A wellness calendar is good for an animal coming out of surgery or in a rehab situation. Put the week you get to go back to the dog park on the calendar! Or the date you can get back in the saddle. Or when the cat gets to go outside again.

One horse trainer hired me because a horse named Calvin was bucking people off regularly—and he was expected to go to a horse show. I sensed that the horse didn't really understand what was expected of him and needed it all laid out clearly and completely. The trainer made a calendar, visible from the horse's stall, that listed everything that had to happen, spelled out by day, such as "Day 30: Practice." As they got closer to the horse show date, the calendar included things like "Day 3: A bath," "Day 2: Braiding," and "Day 1, Trailer ride." The trainer also made a separate calendar for what would happen at the horse show, including what times this horse would be riding. Calvin did very well with this shared and structured information.

Rituals

Speaking of structure, if you do them regularly, rituals bring a sense of structure to the day or week. Some people give a dog or a horse a certain treat after a show. While I'm not a big treat giver, I do take a moment before bed to go to the barn with the dogs to feed the horses and tuck them in, followed by coming back into the house, where the cats line up for their treats and then the dogs get theirs. It's a regular opportunity to say "I love you" to each of them and ponder the day. It gives the household and its many characters a sense of harmony and balance.

Altar

Creating an altar is an amazing way to honor the present situation, respect an animal's need for extra attention, pray publicly, and create a healing or shift in the household. You can include a symbol or a picture of a desired outcome on your altar. You can take photos of your animals when they are at a powerful stage in their life and place them on the altar too. By focusing on them occasionally, you raise your vibration by triggering love hormones, and you can transfer that feeling to them.

Visualization

This is a very powerful technique. If an animal has been ill, visualizing its recovery is very helpful. Many of my clients have used visualization to help their animals recover, and it's a powerful tool for behaviors as well. Picture the behavior you want to see and you'll be creating new neuropathways for something different to happen.

At one point along the way to getting Rollie comfortable with the trailer, I used a powerful visualization that included the feeling of joy and pride for his accomplishment of walking in easily and effortlessly. It did the trick! The very next time I loaded Rollie into the trailer, it was picture perfect. And I was proud of both of us!

In preparation for visualizing, I have my clients take a few moments to fill their auric field with love, so much love that they are practically bursting. I have found this to be a very powerful precursor to the visualization itself.

Pictures

Pictures can be amazing tools. If you Photoshop or cut and paste an image of the outcome you want and place it where you will regularly see it, you can shift the morphic resonance of your household.

Clients of mine with animals that don't get along sometimes take pictures of the animals sleeping and place those photos on a couch. There are your animals peacefully together on the couch. Why is this important? Sleeping is the most relaxed and trusting state an animal can be in; when they're asleep, they trust the universe. Animals sleeping next to each other trust each other.

Place the picture you're using to create a shift in as many locations as it takes for you to view the image often. That way, it will permeate your subconscious, creating neuropathways in your mind that will eventually become a reality in your home. The refrigerator, your desk at home and at work, in the car, and next to the sink where you brush your teeth are all good places to inspire your unconscious mind.

Another helpful picture to use is one of the animal in its prime, as you might use on your altar as well. Whether it's a picture of prime health, behavior, or performance, it's a great way to remind yourself to reflect this picture of confidence and wellness back to your animals.

Vision Boards

This takes visualization and pictures a step further by assembling several images in one place, and it's a great way to inspire yourself to do a little bit more. It is very dreary in the Seattle area where I live, and it's all too easy to talk myself out of riding. That's why I keep a vision board of beautiful dressage riders in the barn to motivate me. I also have a vision board of peaceful horses on the trail to inspire my horse Gabrielle to chill out on the trail!

Guided Imagery

The spoken word is a very powerful tool for creating the outcome you want. I once taught a special animal communication class for kids, a group of young girls who were going out of state for a big horse competition. For part of the class, I created a guided meditation in which they imagined jumping the course perfectly and ended the meditation by imagining the excitement, pride, and sense of accomplishment they would feel at the end of the show. To a girl, they all did very well in the horse show.

Another guided meditation I use is for people whose households are out of balance or chaotic. I have them gather all their energy and bring it back into their center to create a solid sense of themselves. Then I guide them through their home as they replace chaos with harmony. This is especially good when animals aren't getting along in the home.

Goals and Intentions

This one works for health and behavior issues. Having goals and intentions in mind when rehabbing an animal after a surgery or an injury helps keep the end in sight, rather than focusing on setbacks. For improving performance, such as moving up a level in an equestrian sport or a dog show, having goals and intentions focuses your work. It also works for training; when people think they will never get their dog socialized, it is important to focus on that goal instead!

The Law of Expectation

Many of us have had a lot of practice doing this backward: "That dog is just not going to come to you." Or perhaps we get a diagnosis and expect it to be a death sentence. But this works very powerfully in the other direction as well—the positive one. I often show people that if I just wave my hand a certain way, nearly any horse will step aside. With just a slight gesture, I have moved twelve hundred pounds. The worst-case scenario is that I have to poke or prod the horse with maybe five pounds of pressure at the max. Why? Because I expect the animal to move, and even an untrained animal feels that intention. You can apply the law of expectation for wellness, training, and performance. Simply expect the outcome you want.

Structured Play

Structured play is basically training in a fun setting. It's a lifestyle choice as well, in that you choose and expect good behavior and then set yourself up for success and good behavior by playing little tricks and games throughout the day. At dinnertime, for example, the dogs have to sit. They have to wait at the door and let you go out first. You teach them tricks. Animals love to learn and be connected to their humans. Many people don't like the idea of training. But structured play takes the edge off, and it's something you can do all day long.

An entire industry called "natural horsemanship" has been built around this idea. The original term was "horse whispering." Its games and techniques deepen the human-horse bond, giving both confidence as a team and enabling the person to lead. If riding is the goal, all of these attributes hopefully lead to a better relationship under saddle. At the very least, the games are fun and often become their own pursuit because of the connection this "work" creates.

Games like hide and seek are fun for cats, dogs, and horses alike. Animals have fun doing tricks, and this includes all species. Like humans, an animal may be more or less introverted or extroverted. An introverted cat isn't going to come out to play during a dinner party in the same way that an extroverted cat might. Nevertheless, it is always worth training the very curious. Any sort of mind-body connection is great for super smart animals, especially those that live inside or are in a big equestrian facility with limited time to get out and run.

Toy Parade

Toy parade is a super fun to play. It's just like it sounds: pick up a toy and run around the house together—big excitement and big, fun energy. It is not just a fun thing either. You can also use it to divert the energy of your animals when they are in danger. I used it once on the hiking trail when I saw a bear in the distance.

Awards

When training an animal or even helping it heal from illness or injury, it's great to have some sort of award ceremony. At my house when we're learning something new, I give out Most Improved Player awards. Clients of mine have given out awards to their dogs or cats for greatest healing.

I once had a client with a former racehorse that had a very severe injury. He was depressed and not healing. Meanwhile, he lived in a big barn with competitive show horses. I had this client do the Walk of the Roses, as if she and her horse had just won the Kentucky Derby. She walked the injured racehorse right down the barn aisle in front of all of the fancy show horses, and he perked right up. It sped up his healing.

Journaling

If you write in a journal throughout a healing process, you can truly measure an animal's progress. You can follow the ups and downs and see what you did to pull out of a slump. I have my animal communication students keep a journal of all the animals they have talked to and done healings on so that on the days when they doubt their efforts, they can prove to themselves how amazing they are.

Channeling

Sometimes you just don't feel so powerful. At those times if you think of a great healer, trainer, or even rider and channel their energy, sometimes that gives you just the extra push you need to catalyze the healing or performance you desire. A client once asked me to talk to her dog, who was not doing well in the show ring. The dog let me know that his person was shutting down from nervousness when they entered the ring together. It so happened that the woman is a trial attorney, so I had her walk into the show ring with the same swagger she uses in the courtroom. They did better as a team after that change in behavior!

Jobs

Everyone loves to have purpose. Sometimes giving an animal the job of being the heart of the household is enough to help it relax. As with names, you want the job title to suit the desired outcome. Giving a Jack Russell the job of protecting the house is going to make an already "on" dog too high voltage. Give that dog a job like taking care of the kittens or watching the plants and you turn down the live wire. Hunting for bugs, holding down the couch, and protecting the house or new puppy are all reputable jobs.

Archetypes

This is similar to changing names and giving animals a job. My horse Rollie could get pretty wound up, and he's a giant so it was scary. At some point, I asked him to be my knight in shining armor—and that was it. He has protected me since that day. Here are some other ideas that could help in your household:

- Jester
- Entertainer
- Lover
- Caretaker
- Spy

- Guardian
- Sentinel
- Protector
- Senior Executive
- Babysitter
- Baby Girl

Feelings

As I've mentioned before, our feelings can have a huge impact on the household. If we are sad because our animal is older, we're missing out on a golden opportunity for deep connection. I remember the year I was twenty-six—a tough year. My younger sister had died the year before and my then boyfriend noted that I was no fun. He was right. I was a sad Joan. I realized the moment he said this that I didn't want to be sad Joan. Becoming aware of stuck emotions and letting them go can shift an entire household.

■ ■ ■

Sometimes more than one of these creative tools is necessary to heal a physical or behavioral situation. Recently a young girl came to me who was terrified—and that's putting it mildly—of her pony because he bolted. The parents asked me to talk to the pony to find out why he did what he did. It turned out that the young girl had a proclivity toward anxiety, which had created a certain amount of fear for the pony, and he reacted. I mentioned Emotional Freedom Technique to the parents, and they were willing to try it. I used EFT on the horse and the young girl, reviewing the situation until we took the charge out of it. This took several sessions. Meanwhile, the young girl took a couple of riding lessons on a bigger horse to regain her riding confidence, and her pony worked with a trainer on his confidence.

I also suggested that the girl take a picture of her favorite dressage rider and put her face on the rider's face and her pony's face on the horse. The young girl's father did a spectacular job of Photoshopping the young girl and the pony on this famous horse-and-rider team. She and I also taped some guided meditations in which she visualized riding as easily and effortlessly as an Olympic rider. All those creative tools used together have taken the terror out of this young girl, and she and her pony are a team once again.

■ ■ ■

I think that once you get started using the fun tools in this chapter, you'll find yourself using them often, and it will get easier and easier to set the thermostat for interspecies harmony. There is more that you can do from your side of the equation too, making sure that *you're* set for harmony yourself. That's the subject of the next chapter.

12

Energy-Healing Tools
for the Emotional Leader

I include this section in the book because I have seen time and time again that the biggest blocks to our animal companions' natural healing—whether a physical or a behavioral shift—is our own limited belief system. Our belief systems are usually highly organized and supported by substantial "data." Maybe we had an experience that led us to doubt or to lose hope. Maybe we just have plain old fear coursing through our system. Perhaps we're grieving something old and deep and don't recognize it as a pattern that's now running like an operating system for our soul. The only thing we can do then is move our own energy around whatever has us stuck.

When I refer to substantial data, I mean old experiences. Perhaps you just learned your dog has a brain tumor and your uncle died of a brain tumor. In your heart, you believe in miracles, but your mind is fixated on the diagnosis of a brain tumor equaling death. If your animal had surgery or an injury or if your horse is slightly lame, you might not believe the animal will ever be normal. Maybe you have a cat that pees outside the litter box, and you feel you've done everything you can to fix this but don't believe in your core that this will ever change.

If you've had a frightening experience with an aggressive dog or an accident with a horse, you might show up with that animal or another one with a lump in your throat, a tummy full of butterflies, an unstable voice, and too firm a grip on the leash or the reins. If your animal has repeatedly shut down or acted naughty in the show ring, you might feel there is some potential but not really believe success will ever be achieved.

That "little voice in your head" can sabotage your best efforts as well as your animal's. You can light seven candles, sit in lotus position, *Om* with the best of them, and still be hearing, *This will never work!*

For all of these situations and many more I have seen people suffer through, I offer the following methods to break through limiting beliefs. See the Resources section at the end of this book for some leads on more information. You can always find practitioners who are eager to help too.

Animal Communication

As an animal communicator myself, I can honestly say that working with an animal communicator is one of the best things you can do to heal your relationships with your animals. Animal communication is done through telepathy, the transference of pictures, words, and feelings. Animal communication gives the animal a chance to get the story off its chest first, and then the human can have their say. This process alone can shift heaps of energy.

Hopefully, the animal communicator you work with will be well armed with ideas, healing techniques, and tons of resources—including a referral list of other reliable practitioners in various healing fields. But ultimately, the animal communicator will create such a Zen space for you that after the session you'll feel energy has shifted.

Training

Many challenges would be alleviated if more people took training more seriously. A lot of people tell me, "I don't want to break the spirit of my [dog, cat, or horse]." I adamantly and profoundly disagree for the following reasons.

First and foremost, animals have pack/herd/colony/flock/pride rules and hierarchies. They *live by* rules. Rules help define who they are. Rules help them discover purpose. It doesn't break their spirit to have rules—it frees their spirit.

Second, animals need training for their own safety because they live by instinct, not logic. On the other hand, we and much of our modern world live by logic. When we are in true connection with our animals, we have a blend of the two, instinctual behavior and logical direction. Training opens up a dialogue between the two and lets our animals know that there are rules involved when living with humans that aren't instinctual. This is necessary for their survival and safety.

Third, animals' instincts can and do kick in in very unpredictable ways, reactions we don't even see coming. The animal could be afraid of, say, a street singer with a beard and strongly react with the normal behavior for that species when it feels threatened. If you haven't established yourself as the calm and cool emotional leader, everyone could be at risk.

Fourth, when that kind of normal behavior kicks in, animals can become *super strong*. Your training and trustworthiness make you the superhero who can override this enormous burst of energy.

And consider this: if the animal training you've been through hasn't been fun, you haven't found the right trainer. Animals love training, and this includes felines! It gives them a chance to show off how smart they are, how pretty they are, how fast they are, and how much they love to please you. Training should and can be a lot of fun.

Training also prepares you and the animal for some fundamental tasks at the end of their lives. Being able to get your puppy to back up, dancelike, gives you both practice for an essential move when the dog gets older: activating the hind end when its hind legs are weak. Training also helps you get the dog or the cat onto the bed using new steps or a ramp, and training helps you ease an elderly horse over to the stall from the pasture in the winter.

We put humans through at least twelve years of schooling just to create decent citizens. From there, they can elect to study further. How do we expect animals, who crave structure even more than we do, to survive in this world without training?

■ ▪ ■

Now we'll look at some great tools that are just for you, to help you reach that oh-so-healing neutral state of harmony and balance.

EMDR

Eye Movement Desensitization and Reprocessing (EMDR) is a technique that uses bilateral movement to process a deep emotion. This usually involves thinking of an intense emotion while moving the eyes back and forth (bilaterally). EMDR simulates rapid eye movement (REM), the state of sleep when our eyes move rapidly and we are integrating and processing information. EMDR, which was developed to treat post-traumatic stress disorder and has been used for other disorders or conditions, also activates both sides of the brain. I have seen people who have had severe horse accidents get back on their horse, easily and effortlessly—almost miraculously—after using this method.

Bilateral Tapping

This technique is another bilateral method, one that involves tapping each side of the body—almost like patting the body down. You move from right to left, stimulating both sides of the brain and releasing intense emotion. You can also use this to instill feel-good emotions and to come back to a home-base feeling of peace and safety.

Hypnotherapy

Hypnos means "sleep" in Greek. This term was coined in the 1840s to describe what was considered "nervous sleep," when the mind was concentrating while the body was tranquil. The mind doesn't know the difference between reality and imagination, so if your mind is in this sleep-like state yet fully aware, you can shift your reality. Hypnosis is great for easing fears around an aggressive dog as well as fears that your dog will attack someone else or their dog. It can also be perfect for releasing fears around riding and relieving nerves around performance.

OTHER EMOTIONAL-RELEASE SYSTEMS

There are several systems for releasing emotions that either take you into a meditative state or help you ask the right questions to release deep-seated emotions or belief systems:

The Sylva Method is a self-hypnotic meditation that brings the mind into alpha and theta states to create a deep relaxation.

The Sedona Method is a quiet form of meditation. It asks several questions to help release the emotion you are holding on to.

Byron Katie, a teacher of self-inquiry and healing, shares an emotional release system that also involves a series of questions about your state of being.

Neuro-Linguistic Programming (NLP)

This method is like a combination of hypnotherapy and bilateral stimulation. Using NLP, you can program your mind to hold any belief you want. Once you have the new belief installed, you can anchor it using a physical gesture, such as bilateral patting from side to side, to create new neuropathways and thus a new pattern.

Let's say, for example, that you have major anxiety about walking your leash-aggressive dog. You can install a positive thought, create a physical gesture to go along with it, and take your dog for a walk outside with great confidence.

Emotional Freedom Technique (EFT)

EFT works to bring big, triggering emotions down to the point where they're manageable. I have used this technique with owners for everything from fears about their animals, to sadness around the animal dying, to guilt and self-blame for the animal's condition, and much more.

Feng Shui

This is the Chinese art and science of placement and orientation within a space to create harmony between the space and its inhabitants. Feng Shui is thousands of years old and is based on the *bagua*, which is a map of unseen energy forces in the universe. By clearing a space with Feng Shui, you can provide a better energy flow for your animals. The center of the household is known as the Health Center, so just keeping that area clear is an important step. Clearing clutter is always good for lessening the chaos in a household. Feng Shui is a wonderful study and practice for both humans and their animal companions.

The Alexander Technique

Actor Frederick Alexander created the Alexander Technique in the 1800s to enable himself to breathe and speak better on stage. It's a user-friendly approach to the use of our body, based on the idea that we use only the energy a task requires. Many people slump when they sit, for example, or don't hold their heads properly, which wastes energy. Just standing up from a chair requires and expends energy, and once standing, people often continue to slump. This may not sound like an energetic technique, but its power is awesome. It relieves tension too.

Imagine the authority you could command with a naughty leash-pulling dog if you stood correctly. The Alexander Technique is helpful with physical rehab as well, so if you're on a comeback and taking a big dog on a walk, it would be very useful for you. It is excellent for helping equestrians ride correctly and command respect from their horse both in the saddle and on the ground.

Tai Chi

Tai chi is a soft martial art consisting of a series of movements that create a trance-like state of relaxation. It is a moving meditation that is great for emotional release, physical fitness, and stability.

Chi Gong

Chi gong is another moving meditation technique that has its roots in martial arts as well. It is all about cultivating life force energy, a healing technique that promotes physical fitness and aids balance and concentration.

Yoga

Yoga brings together the mental, physical, and spiritual in union with the Divine. The poses bring about stillness as well as a high level of fitness, concentration, healing, and confidence. I cannot say enough about yoga. I frequently do yoga stretching poses with my animals!

Meditation

In a formal sense, meditation is the act of quieting the mind, either as the end result or as a way to connect to the Divine. Whichever approach you take, the benefits of concentration, relaxation, and healing are endless. Scientists have studied meditation for years and found its great benefits in easing illness and stress and improving performance. It greatly benefits a household with beloved animal companions.

Meditation doesn't require sitting on the top of a mountain chanting *Om* until you run out of breath. Meditation can be as simple as being mindful while you're strolling outside with your dog, grooming your cat, riding your horse, cleaning out your birdcage, or even doing the dishes. Like a muscle, it develops with practice. It becomes a state of being and a wonderful place to come home to for all of you. Animals usually love to sit close by when their humans meditate; they'll meditate with you—mine do! What a comforting state of being to attract relaxed animals!

Prayer

Let me also remind you of the simplicity of prayer and how powerful it can be. Sometimes just asking for help in a situation quiets the mind and eases the pain. Prayer can also be a shout-out of gratitude. A grateful heart is an inviting field of energy for our animals to feel safe in. Prayer is a great go-to place when your animals are in great distress. By asking a greater power for help, you are releasing the need to control the situation, and this release creates a little more space for peace and healing.

Spiritual Mind Treatment

This is an affirmative prayer that suggests the situation you want to see is already present. You can speak it out loud on behalf of an animal's health, well-being, or behavioral challenge as if that challenge were in the past. This kind of affirmation invokes the feelings of accomplishment and peace that are experienced when the desired outcome is reached.

This can be very helpful for people who want to see themselves as better, more capable caretakers. It is also wonderful for people who have nerves around performance. Spiritual mind treatments are excellent for people going through major emotional crises. You can use it so that your feelings don't run amok at home and affect your animal companions.

■ ■ ■

Remember: You can use these techniques and methods in combination, and it may take trying a few to heal a situation. Test them to see what works for you and your animal companion. Also remember that each animal in a household is different. The fact that a technique works for one dog doesn't mean another dog will respond in the same way. Keep trying until you hit the perfect solution.

13

Prep Work: Setting Yourself Up for Success

An animal's eyes have the power to speak a great language.
MARTIN BUBER

It's time to take a minute to pat yourself on the back. You've learned a lot about energy healing for animals. Now I want to give you some tips on preparing yourself to actually do the work. We'll cover getting your own energy house in order, establishing a baseline for your animal, and gathering your healing tools.

Getting Oriented: Where Am I?

I don't mean literally when I ask this (right now I'm in Carnation, Washington, at my desk in my office, but that's not important). What I want to ask is, where am I in time and space? How does my body feel? How am I emotionally? How am I mentally? Self-knowledge and assessment help you understand what your boundaries are around energy-healing work. For instance, you may be too tired to give a massage after nine p.m., or the loud music blaring from your teen-age son's room is too distracting for you to concentrate on quiet energy work.

I start every morning asking myself these kinds of assessment questions, before I move the cats off my feet and ask the dogs to scoot over. I do this self-inquiry because I need all of my senses to hover around neutral as best I can by the time I start my work of communicating telepathically with animals to facilitate their healing.

If my body is achy, I ask myself, "Is this my ache?" I know what my baseline was the day before. Maybe I need to do a little work on myself before I can help others; maybe I need to stretch or move my body to get it into a neutral state. If my mind is scattered, I know I need a longer hike or more meditation that morning. Again, it's all about getting back to neutral.

If I'm feeling strong emotions, I ask that same important question: "Are these mine?" If they slip away in response, it's likely I picked those emotions up from someone else, or they were left over from the day before. If the feelings remain present and they are mine, I can address them. I might exercise—big emotions usually lose intensity with exercise. Or I might look for the story attached to the emotion and perhaps journal about it or tap it away using Emotional Freedom Technique.

Healthy habits and routines like these are a good discipline for healing as well as a way to remain self-aware throughout the day.

Sacred Space

A sacred space is a safe place to facilitate healing, and it's something you can create for yourself. It could be a spot in your garden, your living room, or any area that you set up with the intention of safety. You don't need to perform body or energy work with someone else in the room, particularly if you don't feel supported by that person—that can inhibit energy flow. Rather, you want a space where you and your animal companion can be at peace while you work.

In my profession of talking to animals in person, I usually don't get much privacy. I'm in someone's home or yard or in an aisle in a barn. It's not the same as working at home and talking to animals on the phone or working with my own animals. There are ways to adjust though. I frequently just shut my eyes and take the elevator down: I go deep inside myself and tune out the rest of the world. In this way, I take my sacred space with me. So, sacred space doesn't always have to be a specific location. It can be any place where you feel present and able to facilitate healing work from within.

Journaling

I can't say enough about the benefits of journaling. I have kept a journal or a diary since I was six or seven years old. Not only is it useful for measuring your personal growth when you're going through a tumultuous time with a health-challenged animal, but also it is a great way to honor the work you are doing with your animals.

My mare Pet One died after giving birth to Pony Boy, and I was left with an orphaned colt and no way of feeding him except by bottle. I had several charts going during that time, including one for how much goat milk he consumed and one for how much foal formula I used. I even tracked when he pooped. (Did you know a horse poops at least ten to twelve times a day?) These charts came in handy later when Pony Boy was diagnosed with an ulcer. The vet and I could immediately see what had changed and what needed to be shifted.

Keeping track of any treatments you provide while you're bringing an animal back from an injury or a surgery is very important. Most of us keep our veterinarian records. I even keep car maintenance records, as if my vehicle were a pet!

Writing in a journal doesn't have to be daunting, and you don't need a background in poetry to do it. Simply think of it as a tracking device for where you've been, where you'd like to go, and how you're getting there!

Animal Baseline

Knowing your animal's baseline condition is important. This awareness helps you gauge how the animal is responding to your treatments and to modalities performed by other practitioners. Any sort of bodywork stirs up toxins within the system. Sometimes an animal can go through a healing crisis as a result, appearing to get worse right before it gets much, much better. The toxins moving through the system cause part of this, and sometimes it happens because you're breaking up a pattern that has gone on for a long time.

As you assess your animal's condition with the baseline in mind, be aware of what is right in front of you. Is there swelling? Is there heat? Is the animal lethargic? How is its weight?

If you find lameness, is it a short stride stemming from the shoulder? Does this lameness seem to shift throughout the body? Have you taken x-rays? Have you tested all the nerve-challenging conditions that could be short-circuiting the system?

If your horse has a history of colic or your dog has a history of bloat, what were the surrounding conditions when these problems cropped up? Was there a barometric pressure change that day? Did you slip them a treat that you probably shouldn't have? Did they get into food they weren't supposed to eat?

If your animal has a disease, was it on a series of drugs or medications prior to this diagnosis? Were there other toxins in the immediate area that could have tipped the balance? If you observe a behavioral challenge, were there signs leading up to this? Did something drastic change at home? Was this behavior provoked?

Another benefit to journaling is that you can get all this baseline info on paper and don't have to try to hold it all in your memory. You can note it and let it go, relieving your mind of mental loops, guilt, or frustration—all of that wondering why and how, which you can so easily torture yourself with. Use the journal and/or any charts you work up as a place to store that information, so you don't have to carry it around. That alone will take about seventeen pounds of stress off you and your animal companion!

Grounding

Making sure you are grounded is a necessity when it comes to facilitating healing. The more relaxed the animal is, the more easily it can shift back into balance and alignment. If you aren't grounded but instead feel strong emotions, the animal will pick up on your fear, frustration, or sadness via telepathy. That will create more friction than healing.

So take a moment to shake out your hands. Feel the bottoms of your feet—the quickest way to sink right back into your body and one of the best ways I know to ground. If you concentrate on the bottoms of your feet for five to ten breaths, you will quickly relax. If you use another technique for grounding, take those five to ten breaths while you do it. That pause for relaxation can make all the difference.

Intention

It's always good to set an intention for your healing work. This can include an overall objective—like seeing your animal companion happy and healthy—as well as an intention for the present healing session. If you were dealing with a behavioral challenge, you can focus on the behavior you desire. Prayers and mantras can truly enhance and activate your intention.

Visualizing

Create a little movie in your mind that includes your animal companion in perfect health, perfectly recovered, or behaving or performing in a perfect way. Then replay this home movie again and again throughout the day.

The reason this works is that your mind doesn't know the difference between what you've dreamed up and an actual memory; it believes the movie you created is real. This picture of perfection in your mind's eye benefits you and your animal companion in three important ways:

- It creates new neural pathways that have a power of their own.

- Since your animal companion is always tracking your pictures, words, and feelings anyway, seeing your image of it as perfectly healthy and happy renews its hope.

- It gives you hope when you are away from the animal and doubt starts to creep in. Having that movie to refer to will lift your spirit and create an opportunity for healing.

Tools for Your Toolbox

Now we will review some very basic tools for your energy-healing toolbox. Two of these tools can be used for measurement and discernment.

The Pendulum

The pendulum is a wonderful way to get yes/no information, determine dosages, and measure your work. In the 1600s, Galileo Galilei used the pendulum to keep time—it was big technology back then. These days you can get a fancy crystal to use as a pendulum, but really anything you can suspend from a string or cord and that's heavy enough to swing and pivot works fine as a pendulum.

Psychometry is a method of measuring the expressions of the psyche. Natural healer Hannah Kroeger wrote in *The Pendulum Book* that we can measure the psychometric level of objects of any kind—flowers, stones, herbs, animals and parts of animals, the human body and parts of it. Everything is vibration, and the pendulum picks up on these vibrations.

To get started, take the pendulum in one hand and hold it over the other hand to get to know your pendulum a bit. See how it responds to the empty hand. How does it move? Is it moving in circles or straight lines?

Next, find out which movements will indicate yes and no for you. It's easy. Just say to your pendulum, "Show me a yes!" It will swing in a certain way, and it will move differently to say no. Then ask a series of innocuous questions—Do I like Brussels sprouts? Is the sky shocking pink? Is my car black?—questions that have no emotional content. Continue in this way until you see a clear difference between yes and no. For me, yes swings straight in front of me, forward and back, no swings side to side. For some people it's exactly the opposite, and still others get clockwise and counterclockwise movements. Everybody is different so this is worth playing around with.

THE BEFORE AND AFTER PICTURE

When you get started in the healing world, an excellent practice is to run a pendulum over the chakras (or an injured area) to see how the pendulum swings. Usually, clockwise movement means optimum health. Before you actually perform energy work, take notes about the way the pendulum moves. Is it stopping short over a chakra? Is it going backward? Is the pendulum just going back and forth frenetically? At the end of the healing session, retest the chakras or injury with the pendulum. You'll be amazed at the difference!

Muscle Testing

There are many types of muscle testing, but here I will describe two simple ways to do it. If these intrigue you and you wish to learn other, more subtle techniques, there are plenty of good places to learn more about them.

Basically, like the pendulum, muscle testing responds to the "truth" in your field when you pose a question. From the simplest cell to your blood flow to your muscles to your entire field, the yes or no responds the same way for an individual, though it may show up differently, yet consistently, in another. I might ask, "Is my name Joan?" and my field will resonate as a strong yes. If I were to ask, "Is my name Tiki Tiki Tembo?" the untruth would weaken my field, and I'd get a no.

The push/pull sway test is a great way to check this out for yourself. Stand tall, pose the name question, and see whether a yes pulls you forward or pushes you back. For most people, the yes pulls them forward.

From there, you can test products. When you go to the store, pick up the organic lettuce and see if that's what your body needs right now. If you are pushed back, your body doesn't need it. If it pulls you forward, put that lettuce in your cart!

Another interesting test is to put things like chemical wormers and highly toxic cleaners in your field. See how your body responds. You'll quickly discover how strongly our bodies reject these things, though we often expose our animals to them without a thought.

You can also do the push/pull test on behalf of someone else. Hold the green beans at the supermarket in your hand, close your eyes, and ask if your dog needs them. Then act accordingly.

If you have someone with you, hold your arm out to the side and have the other person push against your arm. This isn't a strength test; it's just a way to get a general read. Next, state your real name. Your arm should hold strong. Then make a statement that's false and see how much strength you have. Your arm should weaken.

The applications of muscle testing are practically endless. You can put products in your field and see if your arm is strong or weak. You can ask if your body needs certain treatments or modalities and see what response you get. You can surrogate test by putting one hand on the animal and asking the questions again. In this case, you can also surrogate test by holding products up against the animal and noticing whether your arm is strong or weak.

Protection

We do our best healing work when we clear our mind, body, and emotions and establish a neutral state. Always ensure that you feel protected from whatever might be unlocked in the animal you are working with. Some people like to do a little protection prayer before they start. Others like to bathe themselves in white light. Still others see a waterfall washing over them. People create protection for themselves by creating a sacred space or by simply having the intention to be protected. Some people ask for protection from Archangel Michael. The important thing is to find something that works for you.

What to Look for When You Get Started: Signs of Relaxation

Many energy-healing techniques involve relaxing the animal into the parasympathetic nervous system. The autonomic nervous system controls most of the bodily functions we don't have to think about: our heart, digestion, circulation, the endocrine and reproduction systems, and more. The sympathetic nervous system is about fight-or-flight, while the parasympathetic nervous system is about rest-and-digest, the restful state that is necessary for healing and restoration. Remember the inherent intelligence of all bodies: homeostasis, or balance.

You'll feel good yourself when you relax and offer subtle little touching techniques to your dog, cat, or horse. And you'll soon see telltale signs that you are in fact impacting your animal friend. You are looking for signs of relaxation, signs that the animal has stepped out of fight-or-flight and back into rest-and-digest.

You may notice a change in breathing, licking and chewing, yawning, passing gas, or a softness in the eye. When you know an animal has a lot of armor and isn't giving in easily to the healing, taking nice, big, loud breaths yourself will remind the animal to breathe. You'll find that when a massage or healing session is over, the bathroom is the first place the animal wants to go—just like humans. This is another sign of relaxation.

For dogs, a yawn sends a signal to other dogs (and other beings in the multispecies household) that it's feeling relaxed. In fact, dogs inherently know that yawning will calm them down. A cat will yawn for the same reasons—and also as if to say, "Oh, whatever." For cats, this is actually a form of dominance: "Hey, I am so much more chill than you are!" Cats will also squint at you when they're completely relaxed, though the first time you notice it, you might think you're making that up! Horses yawn repeatedly during a healing or training session to release endorphins, which creates a calming effect on their nervous system.

When a horse does what horse people call "licking and chewing," they're releasing some pressure or tension or dropping their anxiety level down a notch. Licking and chewing during training can also indicate processing a lesson. Dogs and cats do a variation of licking and chewing, swallowing and licking their lips a bit just before a good yawn.

And while it may not be your favorite part of the healing session, a great sign that you're getting into their system and helping them relax is that they pass gas!

Checklist for Your First Session

Now here's a recap of what you need to do before you start an energy-healing session with your animal. By following these steps, you will both prepare yourself for a successful session and get valuable information about your animal's state.

_____ Where am I? Do a self-assessment of your mental, physical, emotional, spiritual reality, and do whatever is necessary to achieve a neutral state.

_____ Create a sacred space, whether that's a physical area reserved for healing or simply a state of mind.

_____ Have your journal ready to go. Make notes before and after each session. You can add observations between sessions as well, whenever you notice a change.

_____ Establish a baseline for the "before picture" prior to the session. What is going on, physically and emotionally, for your animal right now? Has there been a setback? Are you light years ahead of where you were last session?

_____ Ground yourself.

_____ Set your intention for this session, in alignment with your larger objective.

_____ Visualize your larger objective, and take a moment to run an internal movie that shows perfect health or behavior.

_____ Use a pendulum to garner more information, such as from a chakra or an injury.

_____ Muscle test or use the pendulum to figure out the healing priority for this session. Will it be bodywork today? Energy work? A different technology—for example, adding a crystal?

_____ Protect yourself.

This may seem like a lot of steps to you now, but you'll find that it really doesn't take that long to do them—and the benefits for you and your animal companion are huge. You might need this checklist as a reminder now, but with a little practice, these steps will magically become part of your autonomic nervous system, as natural as breathing and blinking.

When It's Time to Cross Over

Before I close this chapter, I want to say that no matter how much energy-healing work you do, at some point it will be time for the animal to leave this life and cross over to the next. This doesn't mean you've done anything wrong. You can't control the outcome. And it doesn't mean the animal lost its battle with the illness or injury. It was simply time.

Were your efforts futile? Absolutely not. Your efforts created a soft place for your companion to land at the end of its days. You offered welcome comfort at a time of great distress. You midwifed a peaceful journey onward to the next life. It is never futile to compassionately care for another.

And you never know ahead of time. Once, when I was living in Florida, I went to meet a new client, Allison, who thought she had to say good-bye to her beloved cat Spencer. When she moved to Florida post-9/11, the adjustment had not been easy for Allison or her cats. In fact, Spencer's brother had crossed over right before their move.

Allison left corporate life behind when she left New York City. She hoped to build a pet-sitting and healing business, but this was proving to be a bigger challenge than she anticipated. And now Spencer had lung cancer.

In that first session, Spencer calmly allowed me to do energy work with him and told me he was open to more healing work. I was happy to oblige and visited regularly for several months to work on Spencer. He was sequestered in his own little room for his sessions, and he loved it. And this work bought Allison and Spencer nearly a full year beyond his vet's sad prognosis. When at last it was time to go, the bonding that Allison, Spencer, and I experienced together in the little healing room was powerful—it was a very beautiful passing. Sometimes that's what an energy-healing session is for.

■ ■ ■

Throughout the book I've sprinkled tips here and there for addressing some common challenges we face with our animal friends. In the book's last chapter, I'll do this a lot more comprehensively, listing the kinds of healing needs I see most frequently and giving you an entire toolkit for each one, spanning everything from what to communicate to the animal to bodywork techniques, nutrition, and flower essences. Add your own intuition and love for your animal to the mix, and you'll be amazed at the healing results.

14

The Energy Healing
for Animals Toolbox

The greatness of a nation and its moral progress
can be judged by the way its animals are treated.

MAHATMA GANDHI

Now it's time to put everything you've learned so far into practice. In this chapter we'll explore specific situations that people with animals encounter all the time from an energetic standpoint, and I'll suggest healing modalities I've seen work wonders in these situations, creating relaxation and peace.

Remember, when you use the suggestions in this chapter and elsewhere in the book, please make sure you also have a great trainer and holistic veterinarian on hand for support. I'm not a trainer, so I can't bring a training perspective to issues like whether a new animal should first meet the other animals in your household on neutral ground, or whether you should bring your children to the shelter or the breeder before selecting a companion to bring home. I'm also not going to assume that you can do all of the things I recommend. I understand that time, money, your human family, emotions, degree of support, and many other things can stand in the way of your following these suggestions through in their entirety. And if I had the opportunity to meet you, I would not judge you for any of those situations. I believe in my heart of hearts that people really do the best they can with what they have. And certainly, if you've gotten this far in the book, it's clear you really care about your animals and will do your best to provide them with a harmonious, healthy household and whatever healing modalities are within your reach.

Another thing to consider is that it may not be appropriate to try everything I suggest for a situation or even more than one thing. A homeopathic veterinarian, for example, will likely want to use homeopathy exclusively and not include any of the other modalities. In cases like this, I advise finding good, trustworthy professionals and following their advice.

Managing vs. Fixing

In some situations, energy healing is more about managing than fixing or healing. This can be true whether your animal is facing an emotional, behavioral, or health challenge. If you are triggered emotionally or feel despondent about being unable to fix your animal, the ideas I offered in the last chapter may be your best bet. They will help you change your perception of the situation, and sometimes that's all you can do!

Common Situations Where Energy Healing Can Work Wonders

As we look at each of the common situations animal guardians face in turn, I'll focus on dogs, cats, and horses, indicating separate approaches for the different species where appropriate. I do want to be honest here about my level of knowledge about birds. They are different hormonally, have different breeding needs, and have a great need for exercise, something that is too often overlooked in our modern caging society. So while general ideas about communication, energy work, training, and holistic veterinary care apply, I recommend checking with an avian veterinarian about bodywork, herbs, homeopathic treatments, nutrition, and vitamins and minerals.

CARING FOR BIRDS

Birds fly over a hundred miles a day for fun! They have a very complex social life, and their breeding calendar truly rules their hormonal system. We need to know that when we cage these beautiful creatures, we change their metabolism, so our bird friends need special attention and care.

Welcoming a New Animal

There is an old saying, "You can only make a first impression once." This holds true for our animal companions. Whether we have a household full of people, other animals, a mixture of people and animals, or it's just us in the home, when we welcome a new animal into the home, it's in transition mode. And so are we! The morphic resonance of the household will be forever transformed when this new energy enters.

Obviously, creating a home or barn that feels welcoming and warm is the best thing we can do. Remember: whether or not it was love at first sight between you and your new animal companion, this is still a stressful time for them. Even if they came from a loving breeder, foster home, or shelter, they will be tense. And there's also a chance that their departure from their last home was traumatic.

Okay, now that that's out of the way, please forget everything I just mentioned because the last thing you need to do is hold them to their backstory. Now's the time to look forward to all the fun ahead!

Your Welcome-Home Energy-Healing Toolkit

Communicate. Communicate how excited you are that they've entered your world, and welcome them. You can tell them this out loud with a calm voice. Share your joy with the others in the house to make this a really memorable moment.

Training. Have a reputable trainer on hand if you're welcoming a new dog.

Holistic Veterinarian. Also bring a trustworthy holistic vet into the picture.

Bodywork. If you start to see signs of tension, keep up the calm verbal communication, and perhaps rub the ears and stroke along the back on the bladder meridian. Imagine you are whisking away all that fear in one big sweep, from the top of their head, through and off the end of their tail. TTouch would be great here.

Energy Technique. Healing Touch for Animals is a wonderful technique to use on all of the members of your personal animal kingdom.

Nutrition. If you don't know your new companion's history, consider cleansing and getting the gut right first. Look at nutrition from the standpoint of your new friend's personality. Feed calming foods to the more wound-up animals and stimulating foods to the more lethargic ones. Always ask your holistic vet about probiotic and/or prebiotic options.

Vitamins and Minerals. A good vitamin and/or mineral supplement (such as Dynamite Relax) is great for immune support. Remember: even a happy change (a loving new home!) is a stress on the immune system. The other animals may feel stress too because their position may have shifted, so don't limit vitamins and minerals to your new pal. Magnesium in particular has a calming effect on the emotions as well as calming the skeletal structure and muscles.

Crystals. Try creating a little "harmony grid" made of crystals or gemstones for the animal's bed or for the main room where it will first stay. You can place a grid around a new horse's stall. Use peridot for transformation, tiger's eye for jealousy, rose quartz for emotional balance, and citrine for esteem.

Herbs. For dogs and cats, adding herbs in a tincture form to their food may be best. For dogs, cats, and horses, the calming herbs to try are valerian and chamomile.

Homeopathy. You can use a round of thuja to clean out any damage from vaccines. If the animal seems to have a nervous tummy, consider pulsatilla or nux vomica.

Essential Oils. Try clary sage to awaken curiosity and bergamot for grounding. Juniper helps purify, and neroli calms the system.

Flower Essences. Use wild rose to ease the transition. If things get really wild, use Bach's Rescue Remedy and red clover for group hysteria.

Use Peacemaker and Self-Esteem by Spirit Essences. My go-to favorite combo for changing chaotic patterns like this is honeysuckle, chestnut bud, and walnut.

Other Tools. Before the animal arrives, you could make an "energetic introduction" to the home and the other members of the household. Prepare the other animals by explaining to them that they will be sharing their home with someone new and excellent! If there is a lead animal, give that animal the role of showing the new member the ropes. If there is a nurturing animal, put it in charge of welcoming.

Moving

Moving is second on the list of human stresses. Some animals have a rough time with this kind of change, while others welcome it. You can certainly set the tone for how it will go for them. If you know *you* are going to be stressed by the move yourself, consider using some tools like exercise and meditation for yourself as well. Make sure you're getting proper nutrition, and you can use any of the calming remedies yourself. No doubt you could use a little help too!

Your Moving Energy-Healing Toolkit

Communicate. I have moved a lot, and that means moving all of my animals a lot! Right off the bat, I walk them through the new location, verbally as well as telepathically. If you talk about moving and keep the image of moving alive, it's less stressful for your animals when the actual boxes come out. By the way, a friend of mine has moved twice recently. The second time the boxes came out for packing, her dog started flipping his toys into one of the boxes she had emptied. He was clearly getting nervous about moving again! His owner talked him through it, telling him that this would be the last move for a long time.

I always pick out the stalls in advance for my horses, whether they're at a big boarding facility or my own home. During one move, Gabrielle was being transported from LA to Seattle and got lost somewhere in between—Bakersfield, I think. I connected with her telepathically and kept sending her pictures of her new stall and the pasture at this particular facility. When I unloaded her off the van, she walked me straight to the new stall!

For dogs and cats, particularly indoor-only cats, talking and walking them through the whole house is reassuring. Tell them where the windows are, where you think the sunny spots will be, and where you will put their toys or litter box. I do all this out loud. Tell your dogs where the dog parks are, what their new walks will be like, and how much fun you will have as two explorers in your new world.

Training. Have a dog trainer ready to go in the new location. Horse people frequently know in advance who the new trainer will be—often someone associated with the new barn. Investigating this in advance makes the transition easier.

Holistic Veterinarian. Set this up in advance too. You don't want to be searching for someone if you have a sudden need for veterinary care.

Bodywork. I recommend massage and TTouch.

Energy Technique. EFT, Healing Touch for Animals, Reiki, Scalar Wave, and even Theta Healing are great energy techniques for both the humans and the animals making this transition.

Nutrition. Horses need probiotics during this time. Make sure they also drink lots of water. In some of my transports, I've actually filled a big tank with water from the last farm, so it is familiar and appealing. Dogs and cats also need fresh water available in transit, and a probiotic and prebiotic are important for them as well.

Vitamins and Minerals. Be sure to continue the usual vitamins and minerals for immune support during this stressful time.

Crystals. Tree agate and hematite are both good ones.

Herbs. Try chamomile and valerian.

Homeopathy. Use aconite. If the animal seems to have a nervous tummy, consider pulsatilla or nux vomica.

Essential Oils. Jasmine, lavender, and vetiver are good when traveling.

Flower Essences. Try chestnut bud, walnut, honeysuckle, Dynamite's Relax, and Bach's Rescue Remedy.

Other Tools. Your attitude makes a big difference. Even if you have some sadness about leaving your old place, make the whole adventure as fun as you can. Avoid feeling guilty if you think you're leaving the perfect place with your companions. Their perfect place is *with you,* and as long as you have their best interest at heart and make accommodations for their lifestyle, they will adjust to the new place.

Remember: when we move, it starts as an idea and becomes an obsession as we nail down all the various details. When our mind gets busy, busy, busy with details, our animals don't see themselves in the mental pictures we're making. That's when they get confused and nervous—not because the boxes are coming out, but because our friends themselves are left out! So be sure to take regular breaks from your obsessive planning to spend time with your animals.

For cats, the process of packing up one household and unpacking into the next can be the biggest, most fun-filled adventure of all. Cats are naturally curious, and each box could give them an entire day of play.

You can make sure your dogs participate in the move by taking them on errands with you. Consider them part of the moving committee.

Horses can be the go-to scouts in a move. I have moved my horses between extremes of climate and altitude and have found it best to move them in the fall or spring, even if they have to move before or after me in order to get used to the new climate. Show horses may be more used to different climates and altitudes, so that may be a non-issue for them, and you can all move at the same time.

Re-Homing

Sometimes the home an animal has been part of is no longer the appropriate place for it, and you need to find it a new one. For a thousand reasons, this can be heartbreaking, yet it can also be very positive if you make sure you deal with all of the emotional aspects involved. The thing that seems to get triggered at a cellular level for everyone in the picture is a sense of failure. It also brings up abandonment issues for both human and animal.

Being able to look honestly at these aspects of re-homing and being resolute in your decision is the best approach. One way to reframe the picture is that you gave it your best and you were simply the place-holder for the perfect home.

Many teenagers outgrow their pony and move on to a horse. While this isn't a case of re-homing because of some kind of failure, it's often still a very sad transition. The child grew up with that pony. This animal companion was part of their learning history. It's frequently felt as the letting go of a family member, and it might be the child's first true experience of loss.

If you clear the emotions as best you can, for both human and animal, you can ease the sense of longing and grief. Instead, you can truly offer the animal an opportunity for a fresh start by reviewing the circumstances with them.

Your Re-Homing Energy-Healing Toolkit

Communicate. Let the animal know how grateful you are for the lessons it taught you. Let it know that you and everyone else in the household, including them, did the best you could.

Training. Training is very important to help build confidence in dogs and horses in this situation. Handing an animal off to a new owner better than you found it is ideal.

Holistic Veterinarian. In particular, ask about Chinese herbs to ease the transition. If the new home is in the same area, the holistic vet may be the one consistent human presence in the animal's life, so do your best to maintain that connection.

Bodywork. Use massage and TTouch.

Energy Technique. The Scalar Wave, Healing Touch for Animals, Reiki, Theta, and even EFT can all calm the emotions.

Nutrition. Keeping the pH balance in the gut is vital to the health of the animal in this kind of transition. Probiotics, aloe, and even apple cider vinegar can be good for this.

Vitamins and Minerals. Keep these up to strengthen the immune system.

Crystals and Gemstones. Try Apache tears for grief, quartz for clarity, and rhodonite for grief.

Herbs. Milk thistle and burdock are both good for the liver and gallbladder—especially important if anger has been involved in the decision to re-home.

Homeopathy. Again, if anger has been a factor or the situation is highly emotional, try belladonna.

Essential Oils. Try jasmine, sweet marjoram, or carrot seed.

Flower Essences. Walnut for support in a period of change, Honeysuckle to release the past, Holly for jealousy among animals, as well as Dynamite's Relax and Bach's Rescue Remedy are all good choices. Spirit Essences is a brand that has specific remedies for bullying and self-esteem if these have been issues between animals in a household.

Other Tools. Emotional Freedom Technique is an excellent choice for both the human and the animal in this situation. You would start out working on the karate chop point, tapping on the meaty point between your wrist and pinky knuckle on the side of your hand, while saying, "Even though this is so (disappointing, sad, frustrating, maddening, or whatever you're feeling), I honor the choices I'm making." Then do one round of tapping through the points for both the animal and you, repeating the name of the emotion throughout. You might even do one round of tapping on the points to address the feeling of failure and another for loss. Then do a round of tapping on being open to the loving new home.

If you have sold a pony because your child has outgrown it, having a ceremony to review the growth and accomplishments the team shared is a wonderful way to ease the sadness.

Stress and Transitions

Humans break up. Humans lose jobs. Humans lose their adult parents. And humans have anxiety. The common thread here is human "stuff." As you know, your human state affects the whole household. It's all too easy for humans to get so wrapped up in their stuff that they don't see the cascading events in the household until the animals get sick or start to act out.

The biggest challenge here is to extricate our animals from the swamp of people stuff without abandoning them. Animals do a lot to help us, but taking on our stuff is crossing the boundary. It's especially important to avoid blaming yourself or burdening yourself further with guilt about involving them in your problems. Their little souls chose to come and be here with you. Now the lesson is to coexist autonomously, with love but not by commingling your challenges.

■ ■ ■

In this section, the toolkit is for the human side of this challenge.

Your Stress-and-Transition Energy-Healing Toolkit

Communicate. The best thing to communicate to your animal companion is that they get to *be* the animal companion and that you will handle your end of the situation yourself.

Bodywork. If you are in a hugely stressful situation, self-nurturing could be the best remedy around. Your animal will see that you're taking care of yourself and will worry less. Maybe you can find a massage therapist who works on both humans and animals!

Energy Technique. The Scalar Wave, Reiki, Theta Healing, and Healing Touch are all great when you're in a stressful situation. If you have experienced trauma, you may elect to do some hypnotherapy, EMDR, and EFT.

If you are going through a painful breakup or a work-related challenge, doing some Feng Shui work in your house or office can help open up the channels to something new. Yoga, tai chi, and meditation would be excellent modalities to pursue. Spiritual Mind treatments, prayer, the Sylvan Mind Method, and Byron Katie's The Work—any of these can help you reframe the picture for yourself.

If your stress or transition is due to a serious horse accident, then EMDR, hypnotherapy, EFT, and the Sylvan Mind Method are awesome. The Alexander Technique will help you retrain the physical body.

Nutrition. A super alkaline diet is helpful.

Vitamins and Minerals. Lots of vitamin C and magnesium!

Crystals. Put a piece of amber in your pocket if you are being drained by a breakup or custody battle. Put it on your desk if you are in a battle with a coworker. Blue lace agate keeps you open to opportunities for something better. Amethyst helps transform the emotional energy.

Herbs. Milk thistle, chamomile, burdock, green tea, and horsetail are all good for supporting the organs at this time. Hawthorn is good for a broken heart.

Homeopathy. Try chamomilla.

Essential Oils. Ylang ylang, neroli, and carrot seed uplift the spirit, while cedar and vetiver can be very grounding.

Flower Essences. Bach's Rescue Remedy, walnut, and aspen can all help.

Other Tools. Hold a vision of your animal in a bubble separated from you. Your home is a place where you get to be autonomous.

Break up painful patterns by doing new and unexpected fun things. This can breathe new life into the whole household. Choose to be the emotional leader of your household. This doesn't require some big alpha stance, and it isn't about denying your feelings. Rather, being an emotional leader is about creating space to process and witness your own healing, while providing a balanced, harmonious home for your animal companions.

Behavioral Issues

Just as humans have their own stuff, animals have theirs. They have their own anxiety. They may not get along with each other. They may be aggressive with other animals in your household, other animals in general, or people. Some animals pee in the house in reaction to something that's happening there. Some have inexplicable fears, especially in response to thunder and other loud noises.

As the emotional leader, you have the opportunity to be causal to their reality!

Because we can't "talk them out of" their emotions in the same way we could logically explain a situation to a child, we have to find other ways to help our animals shift out of their patterns of behavior. The two best ways that I have found to do this are these: offering them something else to do, and getting them back in their bodies. I talked about muscle memory in the first part of the book; this is one of the places where muscle memory really shows itself.

The emotions and behavior you're seeing might be the result of a prior situation. Let's say you have a dog that is aggressive as a result of being attacked when it was young. You could work directly on the behavior, but this is also an important time to reshape the patterns of the body through bodywork and energy healing.

Anxiety can reside in the body like a hidden enemy that eventually has to come out, and when it does—usually triggered by an old memory—animals can be overcome by it. They can get to the point where they might not be able to stop themselves from acting out. Nervous behavior falls into this category as well, including scratching, pulling hair out, digging, and chewing the house apart.

Aggression usually comes from a bad experience, a head injury, or even from the animal's biochemical system being pushed out of whack by something like a thyroid imbalance. Many aggressive dogs have a very tight hind end, as if they're ready to spring forth from behind—again, the emotion finding a way to come up and out.

The fear underlying a behavior problem can come from a variety of sources. A puppy could have been born timid and then was completely run over by the rest of the litter. Something could have happened at a young age that imprinted on the animal. Fear can come from lack of socialization or from abuse or neglect. Usually, it turns the animal inward and can immobilize it.

Depression is a little different. It can come from picking up on their people's stuff, especially if the animal is super empathic. It can also be the result of a long-running period of grief or a transition in their own life, like show dogs or horses retiring and losing their job. Grief in animals is very similar to human grief. The difference is that they can come in and out of it and not be bothered when they snap out of it for a bit. A cat may really enjoy hunting for a few minutes and then walk back into the house and realize its companion isn't there anymore and sink back into grief. Then the next minute, it could be engaged by something else all over again.

Your Behavioral-Issues Energy-Healing Toolkit

Communicate. Leading up to your communication with an animal with behavior issues, it is important for you to get a sense of balance from within. Then communicate about the fun things you and the animal have done and more fun things to come in the future. Keep the focus on the behavior you desire.

Choose your words carefully, remembering that animals don't understand grammar, but they do see the pictures the words represent. If you say, "Don't bite the neighbor's dog," you are actually sending a picture of biting the neighbor's dog! Instead, try, "There's our friend. Oh, what a nice collar!"

Communication with animals that are experiencing anxiety should focus on the present moment, telling them that they are fine and reinforcing in the moment the positive things the future holds. If you're dealing with separation anxiety, don't fall into a common trap of talking about "the forever home." Every time you bring that up, they can wonder, "Why did she say that again?" Instead, focus your communication on the ordinary daily events of life. Say, "I'm going to work." Then do some errands—even if you hate errands. Tell them, "You stay and hold the couch down. Don't let it move!" Or put them in charge of someone else in the house. If you have a single animal, when you leave the house you could say, "I hope this remains a bug-free zone. I am counting on you!"

With animals that experience aggression, it really helps to use upbeat tones and suggest that everyone on the planet is a friend and has equal value. Make the UPS man a friend, the neighbor's dog a friend, and even that squirrel darting across your dog's yard a friend.

Communication with an animal that is fearful should remain mostly in the present moment and then forecast out a bit. Simply say, "You can do it. You are so brave. You are amazing at this stuff." Use solid, upbeat, confident tones, and focus on the desired outcome.

Communication about depression and grief can be done in fewer words. It's best to communicate a sense of peace, so the animal knows it's safe to feel.

Training. With behavior issues, you can't go wrong with training. If the animal has lost its sense of worth due to a job change or a loss of some kind, training gives them something to look forward to in their day. When it comes to anxiety or aggression, training is absolutely necessary. It gives the animal confidence and diverts attention. They can come outside of themselves and into a more positive atmosphere.

Holistic Veterinarian. Working with a holistic veterinarian is also key when behavior is an issue. A whole-food diet that truly feeds the body—and that doesn't add further irritation for the anxious or aggressive animal—is a great help. Think of food as nurturing. Your holistic veterinarian may also have ideas about Chinese herbs to support the animal's whole system.

Bodywork. Anxiety responds to acupuncture, massage, TTouch, and acupressure. Aggression can be helped by the Bowen Technique, myofascial release, chiropractic, acupressure, cranial sacral work, and TTouch. For fear, try TTouch, cranial sacral work, acupressure, or acupuncture to calm the nervous system—make sure you address the whole body. Massage, TTouch, acupressure, and acupuncture are helpful for depression. Massage, TTouch and acupressure will also help ease grief.

Energy Technique. For anxiety, use Healing Touch for Animals, the Scalar Wave, Reiki, Theta, and EFT for animals. Aggression responds to the same modalities—and humans need these too because aggression is traumatizing for everyone. You can use the same techniques for fear, depression, and grief.

Nutrition. Balancing the gut pH is first priority. Balancing the stomach in particular is very important. Some anxiety could even be ulcer related—who knows which came first, the chicken or the egg? Aloe, probiotics, and prebiotics can be given to horses, dogs, and cats.

Second if not equal in priority is balancing the hormonal challenges that happen with stress. Anxiety, aggression, and fear cause what I call "adrenal animals." Look to your green vegetables to feed both dogs' and cats' adrenals. Use broccoli, kale, parsley, and spinach, in addition to carrots. Dynamite has a product called Herbal Greens; sea greens are also good in this situation.

Vitamins and Minerals. Antioxidants and magnesium balance emotions in horses, dogs, and cats. Immune system–building vitamins and minerals help as well; you don't want stress chipping away at the immune system to create another challenge.

Crystals. For anxiety use rose quartz, blue lace agate, angelite, celestite. To invoke a sense in the animal that it is never alone, use rose quartz and chrysalcraze. For aggression, celestial quartz can help uninstall an emotional program. Fear responds to blue topaz and black tourmaline. For a reactive type of fear and to help the animal come out of its shell, try dogtooth calcite, rose quartz, and citrine for esteem. Treat depression with sunstone and tiger's eye, and grief with rose quartz and amethyst.

If the animal has been neglected or abused, add rhodochrosite and watermelon tourmaline for well-being and upliftment. To shift a behavior or pattern, use leopardskin jasper, and to balance the emotions and clear out old patterns, magnesite is a good choice.

Herbs. Chamomile, hops, and vervain promote relaxation. Valerian can act almost like a sedative. If you have a nervous horse, none of these herbs "test" at horse shows. Relaxation is a key component in moving past the challenges of anxiety, aggression, fear, depression, and grief.

Homeopathy. Anxiety responds to nux vomica and aconite. For aggression, stramonium is a great general remedy; use belladonna for a full-on rage attack and lachesis if the aggression stems from jealousy. If there was a head injury, arnica montana is a good choice. Hypericum will help with any nerve damage. Fear of loud noises, fireworks, and thunder and startling easily call for phosphorus and borax. Melatonin is known to help as well. Arsenicum is good for the "'fraidy cat," whether it is a dog, a horse, or a cat. Aconite is a great remedy for animals that have fear from a traumatic experience. Depression and grief respond to ignatia.

Essential Oils. For anxiety use peppermint, juniper, cedarwood, clary sage, bergamot, jasmine, lemon, and rose. Good oils for aggression are frankincense, geranium, myrrh, orange, sandalwood, and ylang ylang. For fear, use bergamot, clary sage, rose, sandalwood, and ylang ylang. Depression responds to basil, clary sage, tangerine, lavender, and ylang ylang, and grief responds to bergamot, Roman chamomile, and eucalyptus.

Flower Essences. For anxiety try heather, honeysuckle, white chestnut, aspen, red chestnut, or olive. Crab apple and cherry plum can

213

be used when grooming or other behaviors become obsessive habits; chestnut bud helps change the pattern. For separation anxiety, use a combination of aspen, mimulus, and larch. Aggression calls for holly or cherry plum. Use vine for the more dominant personality. Fear responds to mimulus, red chestnut, aspen, and rock rose. Depression responds to gentian, hornbeam, wild rose, and willow. For grief, choose gorse or mustard.

Other Tools. Exercise is the first tool; it helps move the energy of all five of these emotional states: anxiety, aggression, fear, depression, and grief. It's also important to be clear about your own levels with these emotions. Can you be objective and rate those feelings on a scale of one to ten, with ten being the highest? If you are anywhere above a six, please consider using the human tools to clear your own field of energy before you work with your animal. If you're inclined to feel guilty or to worry a great deal, you may want to clear these emotions too. An anxious animal feeds off of these feelings, generating more anxiety. The leader of a pride, pack, herd, or flock provides a feeling of safety—that is your job. Now let's look at other tools specific to each emotion.

ANXIETY

- Whether you have a cat, a horse, a dog, a bird, or any other type of animal living in your home, it needs a sense of purpose. The anxious animal needs a job, an archetype, or a superpower that feels heroic.

- Use your own Law of Expectation for a balanced and harmonious household. Create guided imagery of what this looks like, and say it out loud in an affirmation.

- If an animal goes to shows regularly, establishing goals, intentions, and calendars that outline what you expect helps a lot. Place the calendars where you both can see them. Even if the animal boards at a big public barn, you can still have a fun dream board on the stall door or the inside of the tack locker.

- For dogs and cats, create a loving, relaxing ritual as you leave each day. Your own strong feelings of guilt because you are going to work *and* to dinner afterward can compound the animal's sense of worry. Performing a regular ritual before you dash off to work can create a sense of greater ease.

- Create a vision board at work with photos of your animal at peace, as if you had a camera at home and on the monitor you could see your animal companion soundly sleeping. Games are awesome for anxious animals. Natural horsemanship and training a dog or a cat to do tricks are great confidence-building activities for both your animal companion and you.

Here are some species-specific activities: Let herding animals herd—even if that means herding you in your apartment hallway. You can do nose works—a hide-and-sniff game—in a studio apartment, with both dogs and cats. Cats love to hunt, so trail a string behind you and walk through your space. How about taking an anxious colt that will eventually become an endurance horse on a river walk? Take the time to investigate the species- or breed-specific nature of your animal companion, and then create activities to engage that natural spirit.

AGGRESSION

- Many of the same methods for relieving an anxious animal apply here too. I am a fan of giving animals a time-out—a chance to just be. With horses it's a little more difficult, but they know when they're in trouble.

- I cannot stress training enough!

- Creating a hierarchy list is very important with an aggressive animal because you are always at the top of that list, followed by any other humans! Then remind the animal which other animals came into the household first. When you go outside, make it clear that as the leader of the pack, it's your job to protect and care for the animal, not the other way around. Period. End of story.

- If there is aggression between animals at home, training and games are vital. They give the weaker ones a little more confidence and help the more dominant ones feel like they're having special time with you.

- In the case of animal aggression toward humans, if training isn't cutting it, you may want to consider a behaviorist. In many states, one dog bite equals euthanasia. It is your job to keep your animal safe; it's also your job to manage this problem ASAP!

- Managing aggression may mean that your animal companion never leaves your home or yard. Or it could mean liberating your fears and training the animal by working through every underlying issue with a great trainer.

- If your animal is aggressive toward other animals at random or profiles small dogs or cats, these are also very important issues to address immediately to keep your animal (and you) from getting into trouble with the law. Training is absolutely necessary in such cases.

- In all cases of aggression—and especially if you have been hurt or you have seen someone else get hurt—use the human tools like EFT, EMDR, hypnotherapy, and the Sylvan Mind Method. You need to get the past trauma out of your own field of energy. The way you pick up the leash or handle the horse will instantly translate your fear. Your vocal tone and your physical stance will also telegraph fear.

- In addition to working with trainers, behaviorists, horse whisperers, and holistic vets, as odd as this may sound, learning the Alexander Technique can help a lot. That's because you learn how to hold a strong posture, and animals respond to body language that commands their attention.

FEAR

A scared animal goes into fight-or-flight response. Fearful animals also have a tendency to leave their bodies and live in their heads, creating a tunnel-vision flight pattern. When this happens, only the front legs will get them where they want to go; their hind end is a nonissue. This in itself is why a horse can become dangerous when it's afraid—its hind end can swing around as the front end tries to assess the situation. Dogs and cats lower their hind ends, tuck tail, and flee.

The ultimate goal of the tools you use to ease fear is to create a sense of safety and trust in you as the emotional leader. Many of the same creative tools I listed for anxiety and aggression also work for fear. Here are some additional thoughts:

- Body wraps. For animals that are afraid of loud noises like thunder, you can use clothes, "thunder shirts," or Linda Tellington-Jones body wraps. Tellington-Jones created a body wrap technique using a simple Ace bandage. You take the bandage and wrap it around the front end; it crosses over at about the mid-back and wraps back down under the rump yet above the hocks (the backward knee). The end shape is a figure 8—or infinity! The entire body feels embraced, and the animal is reminded of its entire physical being.

- Use the games I mentioned in the anxiety section. This is so important. It engages you with the animal, and for the moment, they're no longer suffocated by their fear.

- Taking the time to just touch them and breathe does wonders. Even if you can't touch your frightened cat, share space, breathe slowly, and blink your eyes slowly; see if the cat will mimic you. See if you can get a big yawn out of your cat!

- Believe it or not, you can do the same with dogs and horses. They love to breathe with you. They love to share space. See if you can get a yawn fest going!

- If you have muscle tested and think that the fears stem from vaccinosis, thuja (a homeopathic remedy) and mimulus (a flower essence) would be great to use in combination with a bodywork like TTouch to reprogram the muscle memory.

DEPRESSION AND GRIEF

Both of these emotions usually make an animal super introspective. Bodywork, activities, and a calendar of things to look forward to will allow the animal to process their emotions while integrating the present moment. Use games and activities to get them to come forward, out of their deep, mysterious, faraway world.

TRAINING AND SHOWING

Both training and showing can create additional stress for your animal companion. Training can add mental stress, while showing adds performance stress. By nature, some animals are built to please, others are "show-offs," and many are competitive. Training and shows can be fine for all these types of animals, but take the time to understand that they create additional stress and use the tools in this book to nurture them through the experience.

The flower essence olive is awesome for the dog or the horse that tends to give too much during training. Red chestnut works for the show animal that overextends and perhaps doesn't ground.

Illness

Sadly, as time goes on, we're seeing more and more people-type illnesses in our animal friends. The list of these illnesses seems endless. I won't be able to go over all of them here, but I can cover a few. Most illnesses have two things in common: the immune system is involved, and the gut is involved. If your animal has an illness that isn't listed here, some of the ideas I present here might spur you into researching holistic approaches for your particular challenge. In the case of laminitis, follow along through the Metabolic Disorders section and look at the lameness list below, under Injuries.

We'll look at these five categories:

> Cancer
> Arthritis
> Metabolic Disorders
> Immune System Disorders
> Allergies

I believe all of these are actually related, and the common thread, again, is the immune system and the gut. Cancers, allergies, metabolic issues, and arthritis can all be helped by supporting the immune system and addressing the metabolic system.

Treating cancer in animals has become its own cottage industry, as the same obscure cancers that show up in humans are now showing up in animals. Put simply, cancer is the ongoing growth of naughty cells.

Arthritis is very common in animals, especially those that do the same repetitive motions over and over—animal athletes and those super "on" animals that tend to overdo it. Any "itis" (inflammation) is a function of the stomach (surprise!) because inflammation anywhere in the system starts there. If the stomach isn't balanced, it leaches calcium from the bones and joints for balance. Arthritis is wear and tear on the cartilage, but you can bring relief by addressing nutrition.

Metabolic disorders include diabetes, Cushing's disease, and insulin resistance. In the case of diabetes, the pancreas short-circuits insulin, which is used to transport sugar into the cells to create energy.

When the insulin fails to do that job, the sugar, in the form of glucose, ends up in the blood, and the excess is excreted in the urine. You will see animals drinking and urinating a lot more. In Cushing's disease, the adrenals release excess cortisol. In some cases, this can be the result of a tumor on the pituitary gland.

Immune system illnesses obviously have to do with a compromised immune system, which can create any of the other illnesses and conditions we're talking about here.

Allergies occur when the animal's immune system has tired and an everyday foreign particle—something the animal is repeatedly exposed to—creates such a buildup that the animal practically explodes with inflammation inside or on the surface of the body. The foreign particle could be dust, a flea, a food, grass, or other substances. The inflammatory reaction could be internal (in the upper respiratory, digestive organs, ears, or eyes), or it could be external (a rash, a hot spot, dermatitis, or hives). Horses have a specific allergy called sweet-itch; it's an allergy to fly saliva.

Your senses get heightened when there is a serious diagnosis. You can go into shock and feel very disoriented. This is the time to use human tools and to keep your guilt and worry in check. Many people blame themselves for not catching an illness in time, and that doesn't help you or your animal.

Your Illness Energy-Healing Toolkit

Communicate. It's hard for our animals to understand exactly how we define illness, but they have much more wisdom about it and know their bodies and limits very well. Communicating to them that their job is to be and stay comfortable is very important. Alpha females and lead mares especially will frequently carry on as usual, which does more harm than good.

If the illness isn't life threatening but involves giving medication, we may need to do some clearing on ourselves. Frequently, we have trouble giving pills because we had one bad experience that we carry in our field and communicate to the animal.

Training. Training can help with giving medications, and it can also be useful in the rehab process.

Holistic Veterinarian. This is the time to consult a holistic veterinarian. All conditions can respond to holistic medicine. A holistic veterinarian may also have a working knowledge of Chinese herbs. In the case of metabolic disorders, a holistic veterinarian may also administer glandulars to balance the pancreas.

Bodywork.

- Cancer—Some practitioners caution against bodywork when cancer is present because the cancer can proliferate.
- Arthritis—Use acupuncture, water massage, myofascial release, chiropractic, cranial sacral work, TTouch, acupressure, or the Bowen Technique.
- Metabolic Disorders—Try acupuncture and massage.
- Immune System Disorders—Use acupuncture, acupressure, massage, and cranial sacral work.
- Allergies—Try acupuncture, acupressure, and massage.

Energy Technique.

- Cancer—Healing Touch, the Scalar Wave, Reiki, Theta Healing, and EFT for animals are all options.
- Arthritis—Try Healing Touch, the Scalar Wave, Reiki, and Theta Healing.
- Metabolic Disorders—Use Healing Touch, the Scalar Wave, Reiki, and Theta.
- Immune System Disorders—Use Healing Touch, the Scalar Wave, Reiki, and Theta.
- Allergies—Healing Touch, the Scalar Wave, Reiki, and Theta are all helpful.

Nutrition. All of these illnesses call for good, clean food: raw meat, bones, and vegetables. Avoid sugars, grains, chemicals, and food with pesticides. Unless you have a great working knowledge of species-specific feeding, work with a nutritionist you trust. Aloe, probiotics, and apple cider vinegar will improve digestion. Juicing vegetables such as carrots, celery, beets, and apples, and pouring the juice over fresh raw meat along with other vegetable supplements is a great plan.

In general, grains aren't widely praised among nutritionists. White rice, for example, binds to the intestinal wall. But when you have an animal that isn't absorbing nutrients, white rice might actually be a good delivery system.

Vitamins and Minerals.

- Cancer—Vitamins A, C, and E, as well as SOD (superoxide dismutase), B complex, and omega-3s
- Arthritis—Antioxidants, SOD, Vitamin C, MSM, and omega-3s
- Metabolic Disorders—Vitamin A, C, and E, SOD, B complex, and chromium (for horses, you might add zinc, and definitely use chromium, cinnamon, and grape seed extract)
- Immune System Disorders—Vitamins A, C, and E, SOD, and B complex
- Allergies—Vitamins A, C, and E, SOD, B complex (for dogs, cats, and horses, also use Dynamite's herbal greens)

Crystals.

- Cancer—Rhodochrosite
- Arthritis—Selenite; hematite is good for calming agitation due to the discomfort; chrysacolla for inflammation—physical, emotional, or mental inflammation
- Metabolic Disorders—Bloodstone, malachite, citrine, atatite, and peridot
- Immune System Disorders—Kambamba jasper
- Allergies—Clear quartz

Herbs.

- Cancer—Garlic, eucalyptus, sage, thyme, and wormwood
- Arthritis—Devil's claw is anti-inflammatory; yucca is a natural steroid. Turmeric is also helpful.
- Horses—Chia seeds
- Metabolic Disorders—Dandelion, blueberry, and ginseng; for diabetes, olive leaf tea; for horses, grape seed extract, cinnamon, and ginger root
- Immune System Disorders and Allergies—Work with a holistic vet on both of these. For topical relief, try salves that have calendula in them. Dynamite has a topical called Wound Salve.

Homeopathy. Cancer, metabolic disorders, and immune system disorders would be best served by a homeopathic veterinarian. For topical treatment of arthritis and allergies, use Dynamite's Release or their Relax. Heel has an ointment called Traumeel.

Essential Oils.

- Cancer—You can put these directly on the tumor: frankincense, grapefruit, and heliochrysum
- Arthritis—Clover, lavender, peppermint, and pine
- Metabolic Disorders—Coriander, dill, eucalyptus, fennel, juniper, and lavender
- Immune System Disorders—Citrus, clove, frankincense, lavender, lemon, oregano, and tea tree
- Allergies—Eucalyptus and lavender

Flower Essences. Finding a reputable flower essence practitioner is recommended for any of these illnesses or conditions. Walnut is helpful with cancer.

Other Tools. All of these illnesses can be treated with certain machines, the Rife Machine and I-Therm in particular. Arthritis can respond to the Acuscope. Cold laser would help with all of these illnesses. Sound therapy would balance the system on an energetic level.

A FIRST AID KIT FOR YOUR ANIMALS

Here are some things to keep handy for a variety of situations that might come up.

- Arnica—A homeopathic remedy for pain, both the gel and the little pellets
- Bentonite clay—Calms tummies, relieves itching, good in a poultice
- Castor oil—Great for swelling and liver packs (which cleanse the liver)
- Charcoal
- Dynamite's First Aid Kit
- Dynamite Trace Minerals—A natural antibiotic and blood cauterizer

- Frozen peas—Pull a bag out of the freezer, and you have a flexible cold pack!
- Solace colloidial silver—A natural antibiotic that can be used in and around the eyes
- Tea tree oil—A natural antibiotic, which penetrates the body quickly for deep healing
- Nux vomica—Aids the stomach

Injury

Whether you're addressing lameness, a spinal injury, a neurological situation, recovery from surgery, or a wound, you're dealing with an element of trauma—trauma to the psyche as well as the physical body. Sometimes this can be a game changer for life. You may or may not have been involved in the actual trauma, but either way, seeing your beloved animal injured can bring up your own old traumas or traumatize you for the first time. Some of the human techniques I've mentioned may be of great support and assistance here.

Because injuries and aging bring with them the probability that you will need to apply rehabilitative measures, you should take care of young, healthy animals now. Help them maintain flexibility, strength, and a healthy weight so that their joints don't have an extra burden at a time of true vulnerability.

Your Injury Energy-Healing Toolkit

Communicate. Communicating in this situation isn't so much about what you say but about conveying a sense of well-being. Always come to the animal's bandage changing, foot soaking, or rehab as if you are there to help. If you need to put on your energetic nurse hat, do so!

Training. Hopefully, you have provided some training in the past, making the animal familiar with taking pills or receiving treatments. If not, bring in a trainer now; they can also help in the rehab process.

Holistic Veterinarian. It is vital to have a great holistic veterinarian on your team to heal from injury.

Bodywork.

- Lameness—Depending on the type of lameness, you might use acupuncture, the Bowen Technique, water therapy, massage, myofascial release, chiropractic, TTouch, cranial sacral work, or acupressure.
- Spinal Injury—Acupuncture, the Bowen Technique, water therapy, massage, myofascial release, chiropractic, TTouch, cranial sacral work, and acupressure are all good options.
- Post Surgery—Depending on the nature of the surgery and the rehab program, you can use acupuncture, the Bowen Technique, water therapy, massage, myofascial release, chiropractic, TTouch, cranial sacral work, or acupressure.
- Wounds—Down the road, after the acute phase, use myofascial release, TTouch, acupuncture, acupressure, possibly cranial sacral work, and eventually chiropractic.

Energy Technique. Lameness, spinal injury, recovery from surgery, and wounds all respond to HTA, the Scalar Wave, Reiki, Theta Healing, and EFT.

Nutrition. Lameness, spinal injury, recovery from surgery, and wounds all require good, clean food, raw meat, bones, and vegetables. Unless you have a great working knowledge of species-specific feeding, work with a nutritionist you trust. Aloe, probiotics, and apple cider vinegar will improve digestion. Juicing vegetables such as carrots, celery, beets, and apples, and then pouring the juice over fresh raw meat along with other vegetables supplements is a good plan.

Vitamins and Minerals. Give antioxidants, MSM, and omega-3s.

Crystals.

- Lameness—Azurite for circulation; septarian for broken bones
- Spinal Injury—Dolomite; labradorite for neurological injury
- Post Surgery—Lapis lazuli; chrysacola for inflammation
- Wounds—Carnelian; chrysacola, blue calcite, and green calcite if there is an emotion attached that has become a habit.

Herbs. Devil's claw (an anti-inflammatory), turmeric, yucca, and valerian are all good choices.

Homeopathy. Work with a homeopathic veterinarian to determine which remedies suit the personality type for optimum healing. Arnica, both topically and internally, is great for healing.

Essential Oils. Try bergamot, eucalyptus, frankincense, juniper, rose, thyme, and vetiver.

Flower Essences. Work with a practitioner and determine the protocol based on the personality of the animal and the personality of the flower essence. Walnut never hurts to facilitate change. Relax and Tranquil from Dynamite are also both good choices. Release from Dynamite relieves pain.

Other Tools. When you're bringing an animal back from any sort of injury, you need to be careful because they're usually excited about getting back out there quickly. They tend to overdo, and then you're back at square one. I always err on the side of caution.

Working with animals to move their limbs laterally helps strengthen the limbs. Horse people all know the move where you turn your horse on its haunches: it pivots on its hind end and uses its front legs in a lateral motion. This opens up the shoulders. Turning the horse on the forehand, getting the hind end to swing around laterally, opens up the hips. Stretching throughout the down period keeps the rest of the body active. I recommend magnets to treat lameness.

Aging

Every animal approaches aging differently. Some love their physical life so much that they opt out at a younger age, not wanting to experience life past their prime—just like some people do. Yet some of our animals age so gracefully that it's truly an honor to care for them. Being mindful every step of the way is the greatest gift we can give them. Rather than viewing each winding-down moment as something sad, perhaps you can see it as a new and different stage, a stage that gives you more opportunities to care for them. After all, they give so much to our lives; here is our chance to give back tirelessly.

Your Aging Energy-Healing Toolkit

Communicate. Any time you review the highlights and fun of an animal's experience with you, you heighten the love and cuddle hormones, which is always a great thing for both of you. The fun you have had and will have should always be communicated.

Training. This is when the years you put into training can really pay off, when you have to adjust how you do things—getting in and out of cars, climbing up the stairs, taking more pills, and getting incontinent animals to stay somewhere other than your bed or even to wear a diaper.

Holistic Veterinarian. Absolutely have one on your team.

Bodywork. Acupuncture, chiropractic, cranial sacral work, myofascial release, and water massage are all helpful.

Energy Technique. Use EFT, HTA, Reiki, the Scalar Wave, and Theta.

Nutrition. Feed your aging animal good, clean food, raw meat, bones, and vegetables. Avoid sugars, grains, chemicals, and food with pesticides. Unless you have a great working knowledge of species-specific feeding, work with a nutritionist you trust. Aloe, probiotics, and apple cider vinegar will improve digestion. Juicing vegetables such as carrots, celery, beets, and apples, and then pouring the juice over fresh raw meat, along with other vegetable supplements, is a good plan. If your animal isn't digesting like it once did, talk to your vet about how bone meal rather than raw bones might help.

Vitamins and Minerals. Give antioxidants, anti-inflammatories, and omega-3s.

Crystals. Stilbite is excellent for brain function.

Herbs. Choose devil's claw, turmeric, valerian, or yucca.

Homeopathy. Work with a homeopathic veterinarian to determine what remedy suits the personality type for optimum comfort.

Essential Oils. Bergamot, eucalyptus, frankincense, juniper, rose, thyme, and vetiver are all good.

Flower Essences. You could always use walnut for change or aspen for fear, if either of those play into the changes of aging, but a person trained in flower essences who knows which essences can best support the animal through the transitions of aging is best. You could also use the flower essences listed for anxiety or depression above.

Other Tools. If your dog isn't jumping on the bed like it used to, there's nothing wrong with lying around on the floor. If your cat doesn't come to bed as quickly as it used to, now is the time to pick it up and carry it to bed. If your horse isn't trotting down the trail quite like before, hand grazing (where you let the horse choose where to go in search of a better bite—literally stopping to smell the daisies and eat them too!) is an amazing way to enjoy some Zen time with your friend.

"Use it or lose it" especially applies when it comes to aging. You want to keep your companion as active as possible without pushing.

Review the Injury section for information about lateral movements of the limbs. This is super helpful.

Stretching keeps the body active. The other thing I would consider for dogs and even cats is to place small objects on the floor for them to step over so that they have to think about using their hind end. Also, backing dogs and cats up opens the back end and uses muscles that would be shortened if the front end were pulling the hind end.

Saying Good-Bye

Your Saying-Good-Bye Energy-Healing Toolkit

Communicate. You don't need a pet psychic to tell you that now is the time to express love in every way you can—through food, ritual, taking joy in the present moment, and all the other little things you do together. These experiences are both heightened and slowed down to the point where they can seem surreal.

Holistic Veterinarian. Yes, bring one in, preferably one who will come to your home if you need assistance there.

Bodywork and Energy Techniques. Use any of the above-mentioned techniques to maintain comfort.

Nutrition. Let them eat cake! This time has to be about joy. Whatever their favorite foods are, go for it!

Vitamins and Minerals. Choose antioxidants and anti-inflammatory supplements.

Crystals. Build a harmony grid using Apache tears and rhodonite.

Herbs. Valerian and chamomile are calming at this time.

Homeopathy. Work with a homeopathic veterinarian who can determine, based on the animal's personality, the best way for this transition to go.

Essential Oils. Choose from bergamot, eucalyptus, frankincense, juniper, rose, thyme, or vetiver.

Flower Essences. Walnut to support the change.

Other Tools. One of the most amazing things you can do is to create a celebration of their life while they are alive, even on the night before they cross over. Pull out the pictures of your favorite times and review all the stages of your animal companion's life. Invite their friends of all species. You can even Skype their friends if they're out of town.

I have seen so many animals hang on for many more days than anyone thought possible. Why is this? It seems like a miracle, right? When we get to the end of an animal's life (or a person's life), we tend to put everything else on hold and move toward pure love. When an animal is being honored with our unconditional love, it's almost intoxicating—for them and for everyone else involved. The whole world slows down into this delicious state of absolute *love*. Because animals are always so present, so here and now, they breathe in that love. Love is all there is, and they can forget they have to go until the body gives that gentle nudge.

No animal can die a minute before or after they are absolutely supposed to leave. We aren't so powerful as to be able to keep them here beyond their capacity to stay. Their ability to hang on may be part of our lesson plan, just as it is part of theirs. So when people around you make judgments about the choices you make at the end of life, just let it wash over you. Allow yourself and your animal the time to be present together in that space of love, or simply be available so you can hear any request for help.

This is all about the co-creation between you, your animal companion, and the Divine. It is none of anyone else's business. You may want the help of an animal communicator, but the day you call one, your animal probably won't be 100 percent ready to go. You know your animal better than anyone, and when he or she is ready to go, you'll hear that voice, whether it's as loud and clear as a trumpeting elephant or a telepathic message that whispers, "I'm ready."

Lost Animals

The hardest thing I deal with as an animal communicator is lost animals. When I do a session with a person and their animal in any other situation, I know I have done my best to help, even if I never hear from them again. Hearing that voice of despair on the phone when someone has lost their beloved is so much worse, because much of the time, there is no closure and all the unresolved feelings are left hanging in the air. The one thing the universe doesn't need is the volcanic eruption of even more unresolved emotions.

Because we animal communicators are so empathic, we really need to brace ourselves in this situation. We need to be the grounded person while the other person is feeling panic, fear, and grief. We need to give whatever helpful information we can about what they might do to find the animal, but mostly, we need to stay steady so that the animal's person can think straight and act in ways that increase the odds of finding the animal.

When someone has lost their animal, my go-to grounding essential oils are bergamot, eucalyptus, frankincense, juniper, rose, thyme, and vetiver. The best practical information I've found is on a website run by an experienced pet detective: missingpetpartnership.org.

■ ■ ■

I'm not a stranger to the heartbreak of losing an animal myself. I lost my cat Alexandria in 2007, a few months before the release of my first book. If I could do those first three days over, I would have hired tracking dogs on day one.

At that point in my life, I had probably reunited over a thousand people with their lost animals, yet for every animal reunion, there are many cases that are never resolved. Although I'm on the high end of success in reuniting lost animals and their people, I still find this to be the most painful part of the job. Here are some first steps you can take that I've seen work again and again for other people.

1. Make flyers.

2. Contact all the vets, pet stores, and grooming outlets in the area.

3. Find a tracker who uses dogs.

4. Get an Amber Alert out; they have them for pets now too.

5. Even if you are an introvert, now is the time to get over that and knock on every door in your neighborhood. You must be a politician, shake hands, and smile— even if you feel awkward. People may not look at the signs you post, but they will remember your love and compassion for your animal if they see an animal that fits your description.

6. Make *neon* signs that will stand out—the brighter colors, the better!

7. Visit missingpetpartnership.org for great tips according to different personality types. For example, a shy indoor cat may not be as far away as you think.

8. Consider hiring a pet detective.

9. Send press releases to the local media.

10. The minute an animal goes missing, assemble a team of people to help you. Get the outreach going, beyond what you can do yourself. In my experience, 89 percent of animals are returned because another human helped.

11. In the case of potential theft, make the animal's disappearance as public as possible to "guilt" the animal free.

12. Visualizing your animal at home is powerful. Let go of the how; it never happens anything like we dream!

One of my many intentions with my program Communication with All Life University is to create superstar animal communicators who specialize in finding lost animals. We are well on our way!

In Closing: Tail's End

As this book draws to a close, I want to thank you for joining me on this journey. It was quite a challenge to pass along to you all the techniques I've successfully used in my twenty years of daily energy-healing work with people and their animals—talk about a memory jog! It is also so exciting for me because now I've had the opportunity to pass all of these powerful healing tools along to you.

In my practice, I keep rediscovering that just when I think I've seen it all, I haven't really. There is always that one remedy, that one idea, that one modality on the tip of my tongue that I think will work for a new situation. I hope that now you too can see that energy healing for animals involves knowledge, discipline, and creativity—all at the same time. With this book and its many concepts, ideas, and options as your guide, I am confident you will intuit the methods that will work for your animal companion. For example, I didn't mention toothaches in the entire book, but if your dog has a toothache, I know you'll find the right thing to try. Think of this book as your companion in working with your animals, there to remind you of all things possible and to be the jumping-off point for you to co-create your life with them. From one emotional leader to another, I'll leave you with this last piece of advice: set your thermostat to harmony!

May you and all the species in your life live in harmony, balance, joy, fun, peace, ease, and laughter! Blessings to you and your animal family!

Appendix:

Working with the Potential Harmony (PH) of Your Household or Barn, by the Chakras

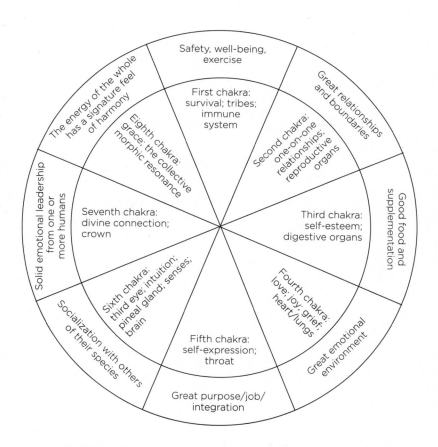

FIGURE 14 The inner circle summarizes the role of each chakra.
The outer circle describes what happens when that chakra is balanced.
You will see I have added an eighth chakra: the morphic resonance of the entire household. All together, this is a snapshot of the potential harmony available to you and your animal friends through energy healing. On the following pages is a summary of the tools you can use to rebalance the chakras.

Energy Healing Solutions for Rebalancing the Chakras

*When Your Animal Is Challenged Behaviorally
or Emotionally*

- **First chakra:** Training, animal communication, essential oils, body work, energy work, exercise

- **Second chakra:** Animal communication, training, exercise, flower essences, TTouch

- **Third chakra:** Animal commuication, training, better diet, supplementation, flower essences

- **Fourth chakra:** Look to the emotional environment—find more joy, human emotional adjustments, flower essences, fun, exercise for all, animal communication, training

- **Fifth chakra:** Animal communication, reframe the picture for the animal, find a new purpose or job or try new disciplines

- **Sixth chakra:** Training, outings

- **Seventh chakra:** Dog/horse training for humans, increase human self-esteem

- **Eighth chakra:** Feng shui, Healing Touch, Scalar Wave, space clearing

When Your Animal Has Health Challenges

- **First chakra:** Immune building supplementation, massage, TTouch, flower essences, energy work, feeding the immune/lymph systems

- **Second chakra:** Cranial sacral work, acupuncture, acupressure, herbs, crystals, machines, Healing Touch, energy work, feeding the elimination center/ reproductive center

- **Third chakra:** Chiropractic, pro/prebiotics, adjusting the diet/digestion, supplementation, homeopathy, feeding the digestion/endocrine systems

- **Fourth chakra:** Acupuncture, flower essences, massage, essential oils, feeding the cardiovascular/ respiratory systems

- **Fifth chakra:** Cranial sacral work, essential oils, adjusting the diet/digestion, herbs, digestive enzymes, feeing the will, redefining purpose

- **Sixth chakra:** Cranial sacral work, essential oils, homeopathy TTouch, feeding the senses, the brain, and the nervous system

- **Seventh chakra:** Cranial sacral work, TTouch, supplementation feeding of the musculoskeletal system, getting a flow through all meridians

- **Eighth chakra:** Energy work, creating a state of grace, feeding and supporting the emotional system of the whole body and environment

Resources

For updates to this list, interviews with experts, and in-depth explorations, visit joanranquet.com.

Books and DVDS

Animal Communication and Telepathy

J. Allen Boone, *Kinship with All Life* (HarperOne, 1976)

Carol Gurney, *The Language of Animals: Seven Steps to Communicating with Animals* (Dell, 2001)

Joan Ranquet, *Communication with All Life: Revelations of an Animal Communicator* (Hay House, 2007)

Michael Roads, *Talking with Nature and Journey into Nature* (HJ Kramer/New World Library, 2003)

Rupert Sheldrake, *Dogs That Know When Their Owners Are Coming Home: Fully Updated and Revised* (Broadway Books, 2001)

Penelope Smith, *Animal Talk: Interspecies Telepathic Communication* (Atria/Beyond Words, 2008)

Marta Williams with Cheryl Schwartz, DVM, *Learning Their Language: Intuitive Communication with Animals and Nature* (New World Library, 2003)

Machaelle Small Wright, *Behaving As If the God in All Life Mattered* (Perelandra, 1997)

Training and Behavior

Sherry Ackerman, *Dressage in the Fourth Dimension* (New World Library, 2008)

Marc Bekoff, *The Animal Manifesto: Six Reasons for Expanding Our Compassion Footprint* (New World Library, 2010)

Marc Bekoff, *The Emotional Lives of Animals: A Leading Scientist Explores Animal Joy, Sorrow, and Empathy—And Why They Matter* (New World Library, 2008)

Buck Brannaman, *The Faraway Horses: The Adventures and Wisdom of One of America's Most Renowned Horsemen* (Lyons Press, 2003)

Buck Brannaman, *Seven Clinics with Buck Brannaman: Complete Set 1–7* (Cedar Creek Productions) DVD

Buck directed by Cindy Meehl (2011; MPI Home Video) DVD

Janet Foy, *Dressage for the Not-So-Perfect Horse: Riding Through the Levels on the Peculiar, Opinionated, Complicated Mounts We All Love* (Trafalgar Square Books, 2012)

Jackson Galaxy, *Cat Daddy: What the World's Most Incorrigible Cat Taught Me about Life, Love, and Coming Clean* (Jeremy P. Tarcher, 2013)

Scot Hansen's HorseThink™, horsethink.com

Penny Lloyd, *Healing Games with Animals & Nature* (Kindle, 2013)

Cesar Milan, *Cesar's Way: The Natural, Everyday Guide to Understanding and Correcting Common Dog Problems* (Three Rivers Press, 2007)

Monty Roberts, *The Man Who Listens to Horses: The Story of a Real Life Horse Whisperer* (Ballantine Books, 2008)

Jane Savoie, *It's Not Just About the Ribbons: It's About Enriching Riding (and Life) with a Winning Attitude* (Trafalgar Square Books, 2008)

Victoria Stilwell, *It's Me or the Dog: How to Have the Perfect Pet* (Hachette Books, 2007)

Linda Tellington-Jones, *Getting in TTouch: Understand and Influence Your Horse's Personality* (Trafalgar Square Books, 1995)

Holistic Veterinarians

Martin Goldstein, DVM, *The Nature of Animal Healing: The Definitive Holistic Medicine Guide to Caring for Your Dog and Cat* (Ballantine Books, 2000)

Donna Kelleher, DVM, *The Last Chance Dog and Other True Stories of Holistic Animal Healing* (Scribner, 2004)

Donna Kelleher, DVM, *The Proof Is in the Poodle: One Veterinarian's Exploration into Healing* (Two Harbors Press, 2012)
Richard Pitcairn and Susan Hubble Pitcairn, *Dr. Pitcairn's Complete Guide to Natural Health for Dogs & Cats* (Rodale Press, 2005)

Bodywork
Jim Masterson, Integrated Equine Performance Bodywork, mastersonmethod.com
Linda Tellington-Jones, *The Tellington TTouch: Caring for Animals with Heart and Hands* (Penguin Books, 2008)

Traditional Chinese Medicine and Acupressure
Cheryl Schwartz, DVM, and Mark Ed. Schwarz, *Four Paws, Five Directions: A Guide to Chinese Medicine for Cats and Dogs* (Celestial Arts, 1996)
Esther Ting and Marianne Jas, *Total Health the Chinese Way* (Da Capo Lifelong Books, 2009)
Nancy Zidonis and Amy Snow, *Acu-Cat: A Guide to Feline Acupressure* (Tallgrass Publishers, 2000)
Nancy Zidonis and Amy Snow, *Acu-Horse: A Guide to Equine Acupressure* (Tallgrass Publishers, 2013)
Nancy Zidonis and Amy Snow, *The Well-Connected Dog: A Guide to Canine Acupressure* (Tallgrass Publishers, 1999)

Energy Books in General
Barbara Brennan, *Hands of Light* (Bantam, 1988)
Rosalyn Bruyere, *Wheels of Light* (Touchstone, 1994)
Master Stephen Co and Eric B. Robins, MD, *The Power of Prana* (Sounds True, 2011)
Donna Eden and David Feinstein, *Energy Medicine* (Jeremy P. Tarcher, 2008)
Dr. Valerie V. Hunt, *Infinite Mind* (Malibu Publishers, 1996)
Margaret Ann Lembo, *Chakra Awakening* (Llewellyn Publications, 2011)
Caroline Myss, *Anatomy of the Spirit* (Harmony, 1997)

Laurel Parnell, *Tapping In: A Step-By-Step Guide to Activating Your Healing Resources Through Bilateral Stimulation* (Sounds True, 2008)

Diane Stein, *Natural Healing for Dogs and Cats* (Crossing Press, 1993)

Nutrition

Jean Hofve and Celeste Yarnall, *Paleo Dog* (Rodale Books, 2014)

Ann Martin, *Foods Pets Die For* (New Sage Press, 2008)

Linda Sanicola, *Linda's Luscious Recipes* (Kindle, 2013)

Linda Sanicola, *Sophie's Scrumptious Treats* (Balboa Press, 2014)

Kymythy Schultze, *Natural Nutrition for Dogs and Cats* (Hay House, 1999)

There are also recipes in the books by Dr. Martin Goldstein and Dr. Richard Pitcairn, noted above in Holistic Veterinarians.

Crystals

Margaret Ann Lembo, *The Angels and Gemstone Guardian Cards* (Findhorn Press, 2014)

Margaret Ann Lembo, *The Essential Guide to Crystals, Minerals, and Stones* (Llewellyn Publications, 2013)

Melody, *Love Is in the Earth* (Earth Love, 1995)

Doreen Virtue and Judith Lukomski, *Crystal Therapy* (Hay House, 2005)

Herbs

Hulda Regehr Clark, *The Cure for All Cancers* (New Century Press, 1993)

Wendy Jennings and Terry Jennings, *Feeding Herbs to Horses* (New Lad Publishing, 2000)

Hanna Kroeger, *Heal Your Life with Home Remedies and Herbs* (Hay House, 1998)

Juliette De Baïracli Levy, *The Complete Herbal Handbook for the Dog and Cat* (Faber and Faber, 1991)

Homeopathy

Don Hamilton, DVM, *Homeopathic Care for Cats and Dogs, Revised Edition* (North Atlantic Books, 2010)

Essential Oils

Nayana Morag, *Essential Oils for Animals* (Off the Leash Press, 2011)

Melissa Shelton, DVM, *The Animal Desk Reference: Essential Oils for Animals* (CreateSpace Independent Publishing, 2012)

Essential oils home study course for animals: frogworks.us

Sound

Lisa Spector and Joshua Leeds, *Through a Cat's Ear: Music for Calming* (Sounds True, 2013) CD

Lisa Spector and Joshua Leeds, *Through a Dog's Ear: Music to Calm Your Canine Companion* (Sounds True, 2008) CD

Flower Essences

Stefan Ball and Judy Ramsell Howard, *Bach Flower Remedies for Animals* (Random House, 2005)

Other Tools

Bradford G. Bentz, VMD, MS, *Understanding Equine Neurological Disorders* (Eclipse Press, 2009)

C. J. Puotinen, *The Encyclopedia of Natural Pet Care* (McGraw-Hill, 2000)

Celeste Yarnall, *The Complete Guide to Holistic Cat Care* (Quarry Books, 2009)

Online and Regional Retail Sources

Communication

Communication with All Life University, founded by Joan Ranquet, is a comprehensive program that teaches participants how to become an animal communicator or energy healer for animals. Ranquet also offers weekend workshops and teleseminars. Learn more at joanranquet.com

Energy Technique

Communication with All Life University offers classes in the Scalar Wave for animals and EFT for both animals and their people. Instruction is offered live in weekend workshops as well as in webinars and teleseminars.

Nutrition

Kymythy R. Schultze, CN, AHI, is a clinical nutritionist and animal health instructor who has been a trailblazer in the field of animal nutrition for over two decades. One of the world's leading experts on nutrition and holistic care for dogs and cats, she is a nutritional consultant for veterinarians, pet companies, and dog and cat lovers alike. Learn more at kymythy.com

You can learn more about prepared raw food at naturalpetpantry.com

Crystals

Joan Ranquet and Margaret Ann Lembo have crystal grid products and general products to help you and your animal align at thecrystalgardenstore.com.

Essential Oils

Essential oils and a home-study course on essential oils for animals can be found at frogworks.us

Other Tools

Pet food ratings can be found at dogfoodadvisor.com.

The Horse's Hoof Magazine, a quarterly online publication dedicated to the barefoot horse owner, covers trimming techniques and barefoot horse care. You will find it at thehorseshoof.com.

An advocate for animal rights, Mary Frizzell is a lawyer by training but an animal communicator by divination. She can assist with legal, political, and ethical questions that may emerge from your particular animal issue or challenge, and she can direct you to additional resources and services in your state. Mary is amazing! You can reach her at maryfaye@hotmail.com.

Energy-Healing Practitioners and Rehab

Holistic Veterinarians

Frank Bousaid, DVM, offers acupuncture and Chinese herbal medicine and can be found at hawcmonroe.com.

Penny Lloyd has twenty-five years in veterinary practice, integrating Western medicine, acupuncture, chiropractic, homeopathy, mind-body medicine, energy healing, and more. Her current practice specializes in the mutual healing potential of the human-animal bond. She is also the author of *Healing Games with Animals & Nature*. You can learn more at blog.connectionthebestmedicine.com.

Cindy Rigg, DVM, provides manual therapies, neuromuscular retraining, cold laser, I-Therm, exercise course work, and nutrition care developed in consultation with your veterinarian. You will find her at cindyriggdvm.com.

Jill Todd, DVM, provides a wealth of services, including certified veterinary chiropractic, acupuncture, and laser work. You will find her at jilltodddvm.com.

Erin Zamzow, DVM, is a holistic veterinarian who provides acupuncture, herbs, I-Therm hyperthermia, and low-level laser therapy. You can learn more at ellensburgholisticanimalwellness.com.

Bodywork

Regan Golob travels the country, teaching bodywork, nutrition, and hoof care. You can learn more about his specialized work at docgolob.com.

Debbie O'Reilly, DC, works with horses, dogs, and cats and can be found at vibrantenergy.com.

Nutrition

Dr. Gabi, a German veterinarian and PhD who works with hair analysis and NLP. You can learn more at equolution.com.

Susan Crawford, DC, works with people, horses, dogs, and cats as a nonforce chiropractor and cranial-sacral practitioner. Learn more at equinenharmony.com.

Jessica Lyman, owner of Traumhof (a five-star dressage training facility) and a distributor for Dynamite Specialty products, offers nutritional guidance and customized feeding protocols for horses. You can learn more at traumhofdressage.com.

Natural Pet Pantry has been providing real food for dogs and cats for thirteen years. They are dedicated to providing appropriate raw and cooked food, prepared locally to ensure the highest quality. People you can actually talk to make the food. Call anytime for a free consultation and learn more at naturalpetpantry.com.

Linda Sanicola is the author of *Linda's Luscious Recipes* and *Sophie's Scrumptious Treats*. Learn more at sophiesshelter.com.

Kymythy R. Schultze, CN, AHI, is a clinical nutritionist and animal health instructor (already listed under Online and Regional Retail Sources). You can learn more about her at kymythy.com.

Vitamins and Minerals

Shannon Myers provides vitamins for cats, dogs, and horses. You can learn more at foryouranimalshealth.com.

Joan Ranquet is a distributor of Dynamite products and an omega-3 with Moxxor. She also offers various Zeolite products, which help with cleansing and balancing the system. Learn more at joanranquet.com.

Crystals

Margaret Ann Lembo is an aromatherapist and the owner of The Crystal Garden, a book store and spiritual center; she has been working with stones and aromatherapy for over thirty years. Learn more at margaretannlembo.com.

Herbs

Frances Cleveland can provide assistance at frogworks.us.

Essential Oils

Frances Cleveland can provide assistance and essential oils. Learn more at frogworks.us.

Margaret Ann Lembo, noted above, can be reached at
thecrystalgarden.com.

Animal Communicators and Energy Healers Who Work Locally and Remotely

Dawn Anderson offers the Scalar Wave, Reiki for horses, and
saddle fitting in the Seattle area. Learn more about her work at
andersonequinecom.

Melissa Bell provides animal communication, Healing Touch for
Animals, Reiki, the Scalar Wave, EFT, and TTouch. Learn more
about her work at melissabellhealing.com.

C. A. Brooks is an animal communicator based in Denver who works
with the Scalar Wave. Learn more about her work at cabrooks.com.

Michelle Bundoc balances the human-animal energy bond with the
Scalar Wave, Reiki, Healing Touch for Animals, EFT, acupressure,
and animal communication. Learn more at aguilaworks.com.

Barbara Candiotti provides animal communication and Reiki and
energy healing, as well as creating custom animal videos and
photo books. Learn more at animalviewpoints.com.

Karen Cleveland provides animal communication, prayer support,
Spiritual Mind Treatments, and animal advocacy. Learn more at
karenclevelandandtheanimals.com.

Willemina De Boer provides animal communication, equine body/
energy work, nutrition, body balancing, Bowen work. Learn more
at celebrationeventcenter.com.

Rose De Dan provides animal communication, Reiki, and
shamanism. Learn more at reikishamanic.com.

Lois De Waard is an animal communicator, Law of Attraction coach, and
Passion Test facilitator. You can learn more at loisdewaard.com.

Pam Finzel provides equine massage, Reiki, sound therapy, crystal
chakra clearing, angel card readings, and mediumship for animals
and their people. Learn more at pettalkbypam.com.

Mary Frizzell provides animal communication. She can be reached at
maryfaye@hotmail.com.

Jennifer Garrepy provides animal communication, Healing Touch, the Scalar Wave, Reiki, and EFT in the Seattle area. Learn more at jennifergarrepyhealingthroughenergy.com.

Diane Garwood provides animal communication, Healing Touch, and Healing Touch for Animals in the Seattle area. Learn more about her work at dianegarwoodhealing.com.

Susan Hamilton provides animal communication, acupressure, and Healing Touch in the Seattle area. Learn more at susan-hamilton.com.

Jane McGrath provides animal communication, treatment massage (LMP), the Scalar Wave, energy balancing, Reiki, and cranial sacral work in the Seattle area. Learn more at janemcgrath.com.

Pam Parker provides animal communication and dog training in the Seattle area. You can learn more at pamparker.biz and theparkercollection.com.

Diedra Petrina is an animal communicator, energy worker, and equine barefoot specialist. Learn more at hoofandup.com.

Joan Ranquet provides animal communication, EFT, Scalar Wave for animals, TTouch and more. Visit joanranquet.com.

Virginia Rhoads provides animal communication, equine-guided life coaching, soul whispering, and TTouch. Learn more at jempecenter.com.

Kate Templeman provides animal communication and uses the Scalar Wave. She can be reached at keltonfarm@gmail.com.

Colleen Twiss provides animal communication and Healing Touch. Learn more about her work at colleentwiss.com.

Kara Udziela provides animal communication and public relations for animal businesses. Learn more about her work at petseyeview.com.

Allison Waldman provides animal communication, animal-calibrated Electro-Acuscope, acupressure, massage, and Theta Healing in southern Florida. Learn more at allisonwaldman.com.

Energy Healing and Support for Humans

C. A. Brooks is an astrologer and intuitive. Learn more about her at cabrooks.com.

Pam Stone Finzel offers mediumship and angel readings. Learn more at
pettalkbypam.com.

The Jempe Center offers equine-guided soul whispering designed to
awaken and strengthen the heart's longing, release disempowering
habits of thought and action, and encourage a physical
embodiment of one's deepest values and intentions. No prior horse
experience is necessary. Learn more at jempecenter.com.

Linda Joy, MSW, HTCP, is a Healing Touch certified practitioner who
works with Donna Eden Energy Medicine and Jin Shin Jyutsu. She
can be reached at Ljoy18@comcast.net.

Shannon Myers is a certified health coach, who provides guidance for
human and animal nutrition, animal communication, the Scalar
Wave, EFT, and Healing Touch. Learn more at feelbetteritseasy.com
and foryouranimalshealth.com.

Radleigh Valentine is a best-selling author of several books on angel tarot.
He is also an angel therapy practitioner, tarot expert, certified medium,
and radio show host. Learn more about him at radleighvalentine.com.

Carol Walker is an intuitive, spiritual midwife, medium, and a medical
intuitive. She can be reached at cjwalker@gmail.com.

Machines

Allison Waldman provides animal-calibrated Electro-Acuscope therapy,
animal acupressure and massage, and Theta Healing in Florida.
Learn more at allisonwaldman.com.

Traumhof is a five-star dressage training facility that offers a Horsegym
2000 treadmill and a Theraplate. Both the treadmill and Theraplate
enhance performance and strengthen tendons, ligaments, and
muscles, as well as providing many other benefits. Learn more at
traumhofdressage.com.

Other

Lost Animal Help: missingpetpartnership.org.
Animal Hospice: ahelpproject.org.

Rehab

Cindy Rigg, DVM, offers manual therapies and neuromuscular
retraining among other treatments. Learn more at cindyriggdvm.com.
Traumhof is the five-star dressage training facility already noted in the
lists above. Learn more at traumhofdressage.com.

Saddle Fitting

Dawn Anderson works in the Seattle area but will travel. Learn more at
andersonequine.com.
Ellen Fitzgerald works in the Denver area but will travel. Learn more at
saddlehands.com.

Classes, Workshops, Seminars, and Programs

Bodywork
Animal Bowen Work: animalbowen.com.
Animal Acupressure: animalacupressure.com.
Cranial Sacral Therapy for Animals: upledger.com.
Massage: Northwest School of Animal Massage; nwsam.com.
Masterson Method: mastersonmethod.com.
Tellington TTouch: ttouch.com.
Water Therapy for Dogs: iaamb.org.
Regan Golob teaches a ten-day program of equine, human, and canine
bodywork, energy work, nutrition, and hoof care. Learn more at
docgolob.com.
Sandy Siegrist teaches a ten-day program to master natural healing
techniques, nutrition, natural horse management, and much more.
Visit perfectanimalhealth.com.

Bowen Technique
Bowen Practitioner Directory

Canine and Feline Dentistry

The Well Animal Institute provides anesthesia-free teeth cleaning
for dogs and cats. Animal guardians are given a report card and
education about what is found in the mouth. The Institute also
offers certification in becoming an anesthesia-free dental hygienist.
Learn more at wellanimalinstitute.com.

Communication

Communication with All Life University offers a comprehensive
program that teaches pet animal communication and energy
healing for animals. Learn more at joanranquet.com.

Energy Technique

Communication with All Life University offers a variety of courses.
Learn more at joanranquet.com.

Healing Touch for Animals offers a variety of courses. Learn more at
healingtouchforanimals.com.

Rose De Dan offers a variety of classes, teleclasses, events, and products.
Learn more at reikishamanic.com.

Machines

Joyce Jackson developed the animal Acuscope/Myopulse Training
and Certification program. Electro-Acuscope and Myopulse are
unique, sophisticated FDA-approved microcurrent instruments that
feature both diagnostic and therapeutic biofeedback technology.
The instruments can locate areas where the electrical patterns in
the body are abnormal and then introduce the appropriate amount
of low-level electrical current into the cells, constantly adjusting
during treatment. The self-repair mechanisms in the body are
activated and healing time is greatly reduced. Animal Therapy
Systems is the exclusive distributor of these instruments, which
have been specifically calibrated to interface with animals' anatomy
as well as their unique metabolism and physiology. Learn more at
animaltherapysystems.com.

Notes

1. Jaak Panksepp, *Affective Neuroscience: The Foundations of Human and Animal Emotions* (New York: Oxford University Press, 1998).

2. Mark Bekoff, *The Emotional Lives of Animals: A Leading Scientist Explores Animal Joy, Sorrow, and Empathy—and Why They Matter* (San Francisco: New World Library, 2010).

3. Richard Pitcairn, *Dr. Pitcairn's Complete Guide to Natural Heath for Dogs & Cats* (Emmaus, PA: Rodale, 2005).

4. Richard Gerber, *Vibrational Medicine: The #1 Handbook of Subtle-Energy Therapies,* (Rochester, VT: Bear and Company, 2001).

Index

Figures are denoted by an "f" following the page number.

D

dandelion, 222

danger, animal sensing of, 32, 33–34

De Dan, Rosa, 251

death of animal, 1, 20–21, 197–98
  animal hospice, 249
  celebration of life, 229
  energy-healing toolkit to prepare for,
    228–30
  grief and, 1, 20–21
  love and, 229
  time for/timing of, 229–30

deer, 35–36

deficiency, 85

dentistry, resources for, 251

depression, 210, 218
  bodywork for, 212, 218
  calendar and, 218
  communication about, 211
  crystals for, 213
  energy techniques for, 212
  essential oils for, 213
  exercise for, 214
  flower essences for, 214, 227
  games and activities for, 218
  homeopathy for, 213

devil's claw, 222, 226, 227

devotion, 48

diabetes, 219–20
  herbs for, 222

diet. See nutrition

digestive problems, third chakra and,
  69

digestive system, 91

dill, 223

Dispenza, Joe, 163

Divine, the, 16–17
  animals' connection to, 79
  connecting to, 185–86
  seventh chakra and, 60, 78–79

Divinity Codes, 17

DNA, 86

dog whisperer, 151

dogs, 41, 42

acupressure for, 111

aggressive behavior in, 23, 46, 64,
  135, 157, 210

biting, 23

chiropractic for, 97–98

crystals for, 145, 147

drinking water for, 204

of earth constitution, 84

EFT for, 162

emotions in, 212

exercise for, 151–52

fear in, 213, 217–18

of fire constitution, 83

food, constant access to, 119

games and activities for, 215

herbs for, 202

herding activities, 215

hypothyroidism in, 74

jing points in, 110, 111

jobs for, 175

leash aggression, 135, 183

magnets and, 153

massage for, 101–2

memory of, 42

of metal constitution, 83

moving and, 204, 205

overactive lifestyle, second chakra
  and, 66

play and, 48–49

probiotics for, 212

raw food for, 120

relaxation rituals for, 215

Scalar Wave for, 157

sensing of danger, 32

sheepherding, 41

short nose canal, essential oils and,
  136

signs of relaxation, 195, 196

stretching, 98

structured play for, 173

tails, communication with, 63–64

territorial marking, 135

third chakra issues, 70–71

training and showing, 218

training for, 180, 204

vestibular disease in, 77

water therapy for, 100

Westminster Dog Show, 55–56

of wood constitution, 83–84

food allergies, 69

food labels, reading, 69, 122

Four Paws, Five Directions (Schwartz), 28

fourth chakra, 60, 71–74
  of animals, 61f, 71f, 72–74
  behavioral or emotional challenges
    and, 236
  characteristics and color, 60, 71–74
  health challenges and, 237
  of humans, 60f, 71–72, 71f

France, Anatole, 11

frankincense, 136, 138, 213, 223, 226,
  227, 229, 230

frequency generator (Rife Machine),
  149

frequency of energy, 13–14
  in energy healing, 15
  of essential oils, 134
  unique to each individual, 13

frozen peas, 224

frustration, 50
  gallbladder and, 69, 70

G
Galileo, 192

gallbladder
  frustration and, 69, 70
  wood (element) and, 83–84

gallbladder meridian, 89

games and activities, 215, 217, 218

Gandhi, Mahatma, 199

garlic, 222

gemstones, 145–48

gentian, 214

geometry, sacred, 17

geranium, 213

Gerber, Richard, 139

ginger root, 222

ginseng, 141, 222

goals and intentions, 172, 214–15

God (or Divine), 16–17, 79, 185–86
  seventh chakra and, 60, 78

Golob, Regan, 250

gorse, 214

Governing Vessel, 89, 161–62

grape seed extract, 222

grapefruit, 223

Great Spirit, 17

green calcite, 225

green tea, 209

green vegetables, 212

grief, 1, 20–21, 218
  in animals, 45, 52, 210, 218
  bodywork for, 212, 218
  calendar and, 218
  communication about, 211
  crystals for, 146, 206, 213
  in elephants, 45
  energy techniques for, 212
  essential oils for, 213
  exercise for, 214
  flower essences for, 214
  games and activities for, 218
  homeopathy for, 213
  lungs and, 72
  neural pathways and, 25

grooming, vibrational, 114

grounding, 190–91

guided imagery, 172, 214

guilt, 162, 183, 205, 208, 214, 215

guilty behavior, 48

gut instincts, 68

H
habits, time required to break, 24–25

Hahnemann, Samuel, 123

hands-on energy-healing techniques,
  95–116
  acupressure, 107–11
  acupuncture, 96, 100–101
  animal massage, 96, 101–3, 102f
  bodywork, 95–105
  Bowen technique, 96, 99
  chiropractic, 96–98
  cranio-sacral therapy, 108, 111–12
  healing touch for animals, 108,
    113–14

J
Jackson, Joyce, 251
jade, 145
jasmine, 204, 207, 213
Jesus, 17, 28
jing, 84, 86
jing points, 63, 110–11
  immune system and, 63, 110
jobs (for animals), 175, 214
journaling, 174, 189, 190
joy, fourth chakra and, 72
juniper, 202, 213, 223, 226, 227, 229, 230

K
K27 points, 72f, 73
Kambamba jasper, 222
Katie, Byron. *See* Byron Katie's emotional release system
kidney disease, 70
kidney meridian, 90
kidneys
  fear and, 69
  jing and, 84, 86
  water element and, 84
kinetic energy, 15
Komitor, Carol, 113
Kroeger, Hannah, 192
kundalini energy, 16, 62

L
labradorite, 225
lameness, 225
lapis lazuli, 225
larch, 214
large intestine meridian, 88, 161
lasers, 151, 223
lavendar, 204, 213, 223
Law of Expectation, 167, 173, 214
laying on of hands, 28
leader of group
  for companion animals, 13, 19, 42

emotional leader, 19, 21, 42, 47, 54–55
  for wild animals, 12–13
ledum, 125
legal resources, 244
lemon, 138, 213, 223
leopardskin jasper, 213
licking and chewing, 195–96
life force energy, 16
limbic system, 134
liver
  anger and, 69, 70
  wood (element) and, 83–84
liver meridian, 89
logic
  allied with emotional leadership, 44, 47
  as human superpower, 37–38, 42, 47
loss (death) of animal. *See* death
lost (missing) animals, 230–32, 249
  pet detective, 230, 231
  steps to take, 231–32
love, 48
  fourth (heart) chakra and, 60, 71–72
lung diseases, fourth chakra and, 72
lung meridian, 88
lungs, grief and, 72
lust, 51
lymphatic system, 91

M
machines. *See* healing machines
magnesite, 213
magnesium
  for behavioral issues, 212
  for stress and transitions, 208
  for welcoming a new animal, 202
magnetic field of earth, 37
magnets, 153
malachite, 146, 222
mantras, 16, 191
massage, 96, 101–3. *See also* touch
  for allergies, 221

for aggression, 212
for aging, 227
for arthritis, 221
at-home techniques, 104–5
for lameness, 225
post surgery, 225
for spinal injury, 225
for wounds, 225
Myoscope, 150
myrrh, 213

N
NAET (Nambudripad's Allergy
Elimination Technique), 152
name of animal, changing, 168
National Association for Holistic
Aromatherapy, 136
natural horsemanship, 173, 215
Natural Nutrition for Dogs and Cats
(Schultze), 118
neck pain/stiffness, fifth chakra and,
74–75
neglect and abuse, crystals for, 213
neroli, 138, 202, 209
nerves, 25–26
nervous system, 91, 195
neural pathways, 24–25
Neuro-Linguistic Programming (NLP),
182
neuroplasticity, 25
new animal, welcoming, 201–3
nictitating membrane, 37
nosodes (vaccines), 128–29
nurturance, fourth chakra and, 60,
71–72
nutrition, 117–22
for aging, 227
for animals, 69–71, 86–87, 117–22
apple cider vinegar, 206, 221, 225,
227
for behavioral issues, 212
books on, 242
considerations when purchasing
animal foods, 118–19

constant access to food, 119
dry food, water needs and, 119
food allergies, 69
food labels, reading, 69, 122
grains in animal food, 69, 87, 221
green vegetables, 212
for horses, 120
for illnesses, 221–22
for injuries, surgery, and wounds,
225
juicing vegetables, 221, 225, 227
mineral levels, 120
most needed foods, 118, 122
for moving, 204
Natural Nutrition for Dogs and Cats
(Schultze), 118
pet food ratings, 244
practitioners, list of, 245–46
probiotics, 202, 204, 206, 212, 221,
225, 227
pyramid model, 118
raw food, 120, 122, 221, 225, 227,
244
for re-homing, 206
resources on, 121–22, 242, 244
for saying good-bye and end-of-life
issues, 228
species-specific diets, 87, 118, 120
for stress and transitions, 208
TCM approach to, 86–87
third chakra and, 69–70
water needs, 119, 204
welcoming a new animal, 202
white rice, 221–22
whole-food diet, 212
nux vomica, 126, 202, 204, 213, 224

O
O'Connor, Caitlin, 34
oil, anointing with, 28
olive, 213, 218
olive leaf tea, 222
Om, 148–49, 185
omega-3s, 222, 225
One Mind, 17, 40–41
one-on-one relationships, second
chakra and, 67

About the Author

Joan Ranquet is an animal communicator, marine naturalist, public speaker, founder of Communication With All Life University, and author of *Communication With All Life: Revelations of an Animal Communicator* (Hay House, 2007). Joan conducts private healing sessions, teaches through teleseminars and weekend workshops, and guides people on animal communication and wildlife trips.

Joan has worked with thousands of individual pet owners, as well as dog, cat, and horse trainers, barn managers, and veterinarians. She troubleshoots behavioral and medical issues, stimulates healing in conjunction with conventional treatment, and helps clients deepen their ability to care for—and understand—their animals.

She speaks all over the United States on animal communication, human/animal relationships, energy healing, and marine wildlife. Joan also donates her time to help rescue and rehab organizations, as well as therapeutic riding centers.

In media, Joan has been featured in *The Hollywood Reporter* and in local Seattle news programs. She was chosen by MSN as one of the "Top 25 People Who Do What They Love" and has been featured in dozens of media including Animal Planet, "Pet Nation" on *Dateline*, the *Today* show, *Good Morning America*, *National Enquirer*, *Los Angeles Times*, *Sun Sentinel*, and Palm Beach Post. She was the "celebrity animal communicator" in a documentary that aired on AMC.

After attending Stephens College, she received a BFA in theater. She has been working with animals for as long as she can remember and is a lifelong equestrian. Joan lives with her large animal family: horses, dogs, and cats.

About Sounds True

Sounds True is a multimedia publisher whose mission is to inspire and support personal transformation and spiritual awakening. Founded in 1985 and located in Boulder, Colorado, we work with many of the leading spiritual teachers, thinkers, healers, and visionary artists of our time. We strive with every title to preserve the essential "living wisdom" of the author or artist. It is our goal to create products that not only provide information to a reader or listener, but that also embody the quality of a wisdom transmission.

For those seeking genuine transformation, Sounds True is your trusted partner. At SoundsTrue.com you will find a wealth of free resources to support your journey, including exclusive weekly audio interviews, free downloads, interactive learning tools, and other special savings on all our titles.

To learn more, please visit SoundsTrue.com/freegifts or call us toll-free at 800-333-9185.

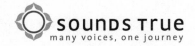